NUTRITIONAL REQUIREMENTS OF INFANTS AND YOUNG CHILDREN

Practical Guidelines

Edited by

Joyce M. Thompson

Nutrition and Dietetic Manager, Angus NHS Trust

Researched and compiled by

Gillian Howard

Community Dietitian, Angus NHS Trust

**Blackwell
Science**

© 1998 by
Blackwell Science Ltd
Editorial Offices:
Osney Mead, Oxford OX2 0EL
25 John Street, London WC1N 2BL
23 Ainslie Place, Edinburgh EH3 6AJ
350 Main Street, Malden
  MA 02148 5018, USA
54 University Street, Carlton
  Victoria 3053, Australia

Other Editorial Offices:

Blackwell Wissenschafts-Verlag GmbH
Kurfürstendamm 57
10707 Berlin, Germany

Blackwell Science KK
MG Kodenmacho Building
7–10 Kodenmacho Nihombashi
Chuo-ku, Tokyo 104, Japan

First published 1998

Set in 10.5/13pt Sabon
by DP Photosetting, Aylesbury, Bucks
Printed and bound in Great Britain by
MPG Books Limited, Bodmin, Cornwall

The Blackwell Science logo is a trade mark of
Blackwell Science Ltd, registered at the
United Kingdom Trade Marks Registry

DISTRIBUTORS

Marston Book Services Ltd
PO Box 269
Abingdon
Oxon OX14 4YN
(*Orders:* Tel: 01235 465500
        Fax: 01235 465555)

USA
Blackwell Science, Inc.
Commerce Place
350 Main Street
Malden, MA 02148 5018
(*Orders:* Tel: 800 759 6102
        617 388 8250
        Fax: 617 388 8255)

Canada
Copp Clark Professional
200 Adelaide Street West, 3rd Floor
Toronto, Ontario M5H 1W7
(*Orders:* Tel: 416 597-1616
        800 815 9417
        Fax: 416 597 1617)

Australia
Blackwell Science Pty Ltd
54 University Street
Carlton, Victoria 3053
(*Orders:* Tel: 03 9347 0300
        Fax: 03 9347 5001)

A catalogue record for this title is available
from the British Library

ISBN 0-632-04891-3

Library of Congress
Cataloging-in-Publication Data
Nutritional requirements of infants and
    young children: practical guidelines/edited
    by Joyce M. Thompson; researched and
    compiled by Gillian Howard.
      p. cm.
      Includes bibliographical references and
    index.
      ISBN 0-632-04891-3
      1. Children—Nutrition. 2. Infants—
    Nutrition. 3. Children—Nutrition—
    Requirements. 4. Infants—Nutrition—
    Requirements.
      I. Thompson, Joyce M. II. Howard,
    Gillian.
      [DNLM: 1. Nutritional
    Requirements—in infancy & childhood.
    2. Infant Nutrition. QU 145 N97842
    1997]
    RJ206.N825 1997
    613.2'083—dc21
    DNLM/DLC
    for Library of Congress   97-22822
                                        CIP

NUTRITIONAL REQUIREMENTS OF INFANTS AND YOUNG CHILDREN

Practical Guidelines

Contents

Foreword   xi
Acknowledgements   xiii
List of abbreviations   xvii
Introduction   xix
  Aims   xix
  Objectives   xix

Section 1   The First Twelve Months

1 Breastfeeding   3
  1.1 Composition of human milk   3
  1.2 Nutritional characteristics of mature milk 4
  1.3 Non-nutritional components of breast milk   6
  1.4 Milk production   6
  1.5 Advantages of breastfeeding   8
  1.6 Trends in breastfeeding   8
  1.7 Maternal diet   10
  1.8 Factors found helpful to breastfeeding   15
  1.9 Factors found unhelpful to breastfeeding   15
  1.10 Failure to thrive at the breast   16
  1.11 Changing from breast to bottle feeding   17
  1.12 Contraindications to breastfeeding   18
  1.13 Promotion of breastfeeding   18

2 Bottle Feeding   20
  2.1 Trends in bottle feeding   20
  2.2 Infant milks   21
  2.3 Preparation of feeds   24
  2.4 Microwaves   25
  2.5 Infant milk marketing   25

3 Problem Solving   27
  3.1 Constipation   27
  3.2 Posseting (gastro-oesophageal reflux)   28
  3.3 Colic   29
  3.4 Vitamins   30

4 Growth **32**
  4.1 Importance of good growth in infancy 32
  4.2 Growth monitoring 32
  4.3 Specific measurements 34
  4.4 Failure to thrive 35

5 Pre-term and Low Birth Weight Infants **38**
  5.1 Classification 38
  5.2 Nutrient needs 38
  5.3 Early feeding of low birth weight infants 39
  5.4 Management of low birth weight infants in
     the community 40

6 Weaning **44**
  6.1 Introduction 44
  6.2 Reasons for weaning 44
  6.3 Age of weaning 45
  6.4 Practical points about weaning 47
  6.5 The first stage: 4–6 months 48
  6.6 The second stage: 6–9 months 53
  6.7 The third stage: 9–12 months 56
  6.8 Drinks during weaning 57
  6.9 Vegetarian weaning 57
  6.10 What constitutes a nutritionally adequate
      weaning diet? 59

7 Iron Nutrition in Infancy **61**
  7.1 Importance of iron in the weaning diet 61
  7.2 Prevalence of iron deficiency 61
  7.3 Iron absorption 63
  7.4 Sources of iron in the weaning diet 64
  7.5 Practical questions 66

8 Cow's Milk and Other Milks **69**
  8.1 Cow's milk 69
  8.2 Follow-on milk 73
  8.3 Goat's milk 74
  8.4 Ewe's milk 74
  8.5 Soya infant formula 75
  8.6 Soya 'milk' 76
  8.7 Role of milk in the weaning diet 77

9   **Food Intolerance and Allergy**   78
    9.1   Definitions   78
    9.2   Reactions to food   79
    9.3   Foods causing intolerant reactions   79
    9.4   Prevalence   79
    9.5   Symptoms   80
    9.6   Diagnosis   81
    9.7   Risk factors for the development of allergies   81
    9.8   Cow's milk intolerance   83

10 **Dental Health**   88
    10.1 Introduction   88
    10.2 The prevalence of dental caries   88
    10.3 The process of dental caries   89
    10.4 Factors influencing the risk of dental caries   89
    10.5 Dietary sugars in infancy   91
    10.6 Preserving the primary dentition   98
    10.7 Teething   98
    10.8 Summary of dental health advice   98

11 **Food Safety**   99
    11.1 Causes of food poisoning   99
    11.2 Reducing risk of food poisoning   100
    11.3 Common questions   103
    11.4 Common food poisoning bacteria   105
    11.5 Summary   108
    References and Further Reading for Section 1   109

Section 2   One to Three Years

12 **Nutritional Requirements 1–3 years**   119
    12.1 Introduction   119
    12.2 Nutrient needs   119
    12.3 Dietary reference values   121
    12.4 Meeting nutrient needs   123

13 **Assessing Dietary Adequacy**   125
    13.1 Risk factors for dietary inadequacy   126
    13.2 Growth and wellbeing   127
    13.3 Dietary composition   127
    13.4 Individual nutrients   130

14 **Eating for Future Health**   **136**
   14.1 Fat   137
   14.2 Fibre   137
   14.3 Sugar   139
   14.4 Salt   140
   14.5 Summary   142

15 **Meal Time Considerations**   **143**
   15.1 Feeding development   143
   15.2 Meal time environment   145
   15.3 Food appeal   145
   15.4 Eating location   146
   15.5 Food as an activity   148

16 **Feeding Problems**   **149**
   16.1 Food refusal   149
   16.2 Other food-related problems   154

17 **Other Common Concerns**   **157**
   17.1 Toddler diarrhoea   157
   17.2 Constipation   158
   17.3 Supplementary government vitamins   160
   17.4 Hyperactivity   162

18 **Vegetarian and Ethnic Minority Diets**   **163**
   18.1 Introduction   163
   18.2 Vegetarian and vegan diets   163
   18.3 Asian diets   168
   18.4 Afro-Caribbean diets   171
   18.5 Other ethnic groups   172
   References and Further Reading for Section 2   **174**

Section 3 Three to Five Years

19 **The Healthy Pre-School Diet**   **179**
   19.1 Nutrient needs   179
   19.2 Healthy eating habits   181
   19.3 Eating patterns and dental health   184
   19.4 Summary   186

20	**Poverty and Nutrition**	**187**
	20.1 Characteristics of low income diet	187
	20.2 Constraints to healthy eating	188
	20.3 Tackling common problems	190
	20.4 Summary	194
21	**Feeding Problems**	**196**
	21.1 Food fads	196
	21.2 Refusal to eat meat	199
	21.3 Refusal to eat vegetables	200
	21.4 Refusal to drink milk	201
	21.5 Summary	201
22	**Obesity**	**202**
	22.1 Definitions	202
	22.2 Assessment	202
	22.3 Adiposity during childhood	203
	22.4 Causes of obesity	203
	22.5 Consequences of childhood obesity	205
	22.6 Prevention of obesity	205
	22.7 Management of early childhood obesity	205
	22.8 Summary	209
23	**Meals and Snacks**	**210**
	23.1 Breakfast	210
	23.2 Meals	212
	23.3 Snacks	215
	23.4 Drinks	217
24	**Additives**	**219**
	24.1 The E number system	220
	24.2 Additives and young children	220
	24.3 Adverse reactions to additives	220
	24.4 Summary	224
	References and Further Reading for Section 3	225

Appendices

Appendix I: The Cycle of Ill Health	**231**
Appendix II: Dietary References Values for the Under Fives	**232**
Appendix III: Welfare Food Scheme	**233**

Resources

Recommended Reading   **237**
  Specific Reports   **237**
    Early diet   237
    Nutrient intakes   237
    Growth   237
    Knowledge   237
    Iron deficiency   238
    Asian   238
    Low income   238
    Dental health   238
    Food allergy/intolerance   239
  General Publications   **239**
    Books   239
    Reports   240
    Briefing papers   240
    Magazines/journals   241
  Resource List: Organisations   **242**
  Information Recommended for Patients   **244**
    Leaflets   244
    Books   245

Index   246

Foreword

It is now clear that nutrition in the early years of life is a major determinant of the growth, health and development of the child, and it also influences adult health. Infants and young children who do not grow in accordance with expectations based on population norms, are described as failing to thrive. Although the first sign of failure to thrive is a declining rate of weight gain, later the rate of gain in length becomes less than expected and the rate of gain in head circumference also declines. Cognitive deficit is a feature of more severe and prolonged failure to thrive. Social, clinical and psychological factors may all contribute to a child's failure to thrive. Energy and nutrient intakes may be inadequate because of inappropriate diets due, for instance, to prolonged reliance on milk alone or because the diet contains too much bulky low energy food. In other circumstances, young children may consume snacks and large volumes of dilute juices which reduce the appetite for more nutrient dense foods. Specific nutrient deficiency states such as iron deficiency may in turn affect appetite, intellect and response to infections.

Feeding and behavioural problems may be significant determinants of a child's failure to thrive. Mothers and other carers differ in their skills in overcoming eating problems. When a mother is disinterested in her child or is herself indifferent to food or is repelled by 'messy' food, or if she is determined to establish control of the child's eating patterns with resulting conflict, the outcome is likely to be that less food is consumed by the child.

Recent epidemiological studies have identified factors reflecting nutritional status in fetal life and infancy which appear to be linked with adult health. Thus, rates of ischaemic heart disease and stroke, and the associated conditions hypertension and non-insulin dependent diabetes in groups of middle aged and older men, correlate closely with lower rates of growth and development during fetal life and infancy. Periods of nutritional inadequacy in early life might prevent the development of new blood vessels needed to allow specific body organs and tissues to develop to their full potential. Specific nutrient deficiencies such as fatty acid deficiencies during early life might affect the membranes of developing brain cells and interfere with processes essential for normal learning in infancy and early childhood.

These are just some facets which highlight the importance of ensuring good nutrition for the young members of our society. The practical guidelines for health professionals produced by Miss Joyce Thompson and her colleagues are founded on sound underlying principles and provide an excellent basis for the acquisition of appropriate knowledge. They also provide a practical approach to helping parents understand normal feeding practices as well as helping them cope with many of the illnesses which affect the young and their nutrition.

Professor F. Cockburn
Department of Child Health
Royal Hospital for Sick Children
Yorkhill, Glasgow, G3 8SJ

Acknowledgements

It will be appreciated that such a comprehensive text has involved the assistance of many people and their help is gratefully acknowledged.

First and foremost I must thank Gillian Howard, Community Dietitian, who joined the department in April 1994 to undertake this two year project. The range and depth of this book is a tribute to the dedication, methodical approach, determination and positive support which Gilllian brought to the project. I believe that she has succeeded in presenting current information in a practical and accessible format and has dealt with contentious issues in a balanced way. Every topic was thoroughly researched and expert advice sought for all sections of the book throughout its development.

I am particularly grateful to the Angus NHS Trust health visitors who provided the main focus for determining which nutrition topics should be covered and the format in which they should be presented. They were involved throughout the project in group discussions and training programmes as well as the piloting and evaluating of the text. Thanks go also to Mrs Jessie Hayes (Community Manager), Mrs Jean Cruickshank and Mrs Heather Goudie (Locality Managers) and Mrs Jean McGuinn (Clinical Nurse Manager) for their support of the work. Our special thanks go to all the Angus NHS Trust health visitors who were with the Trust from 1994 to 1996.

There is a long list of experts to whom I am most grateful for their invaluable advice and opinions and who gave so generously of their precious time to support this project. Special thanks go to Dr J. Stewart Forsyth (Consultant Paediatrician) and to Mrs Andrea Wilson and Mrs Clare McLeish (Paediatric Dietitians at Ninewells Hospital, Dundee); to Mrs Margaret Moss (Chief Dietitian at Raigmore Hospital, Inverness), Mrs Gill Moore (Community Paediatric Dietitian, Shielfield Health Centre, Newcastle-upon-Tyne), Mrs Cathy Webb (Paediatric Dietitian, Wrexham Mallor Hospital, N. Wales) and Mrs Jane Gray (Midwife from Liverpool). I must also thank Mrs Aileen Logie (Dentist at Brechin Health Centre) and Ms Rhona Greig (Dental Hygienist, Abbey Health Centre, Arbroath); Mrs Christine Russell (Head of Nutrition, Cow & Gate), Mrs Linda McGrath (Community

Dietitian, Perth) and Dr Lynda Morton (General Practitioner, Carnoustie) for their help.

I am indebted to the Angus NHS Trust dietetic staff for their support and help throughout the preparation of the text, particularly Mrs Linda Grieve, Mrs Juliet Miller and Mrs Rhona Peters, as well as the secretarial expertise of Mrs Mary Paton. I also acknowledge with thanks the support and expertise of Dr Tim Gill (The Post-Graduate Nutrition & Dietetic Centre at the Rowett Research Institute, Aberdeen) and the invaluable desk-top publishing and editing services of Mrs Jean James.

Many of the above individuals also assisted with a review of the final draft of the book before it went to press, and additional thanks go to the following who also took part in this final stage of the project:

Mr Craig Anderson, Environmental Health Officer, Food & Safety Section, Angus District Council

Dr Caroline Bolton-Smith, Senior Lecturer in Nutrition, University of Dundee, Ninewells Hospital, Dundee

Mrs Sally Bonnar, Consultant Psychiatrist, Dundee

Mrs Brenda Clark, Chief Paediatric Dietitian, Royal Hospital for Sick Children, Yorkhill, Glasgow

Mrs Kathy Cowbrough, Scottish Community Nutrition Group (Chair) and Nutrition Consultant

Ms Tazmina Crisp, Dietitian, Newcastle-upon-Tyne

Dr Morag Curnow, Senior Dental Officer, Perth & Kinross NHS Trust

Mrs Helen Grossi, Paediatric Dietitian, Ninewells Hospital, Dundee

Mrs Judith Hendry, Dietetic Manager, Community Dietetic Department, Aberdeen

Mrs Anne Laidlaw, Health Visitor, East & Midlothian NHS Trust

Miss Sheena Laing, Chief Paediatric Dietitian, Edinburgh Sick Children's NHS Trust

Dr D. Parratt, Senior Lecturer, Medical Microbiology, Dundee

Miss Kathleen Ross, Paediatric Dietitian, Aberdeen Royal Hospitals NHS Trust

Miss Marjory Thomson, Chief Dietitian, East & Midlothian NHS Trust

Mrs Ruth Webber, Community Paediatric Dietitian, Grampian Healthcare NHS Trust

Mrs Julia Whitehead, Research Dietitian, Rowett Research Institute, Aberdeen

Miss Anne Woodcock, Senior Health Promotion Officer (Nutrition), Tayside Health Promotion Centre

Finally, I gratefully acknowledge the financial support and co-operation from Cow & Gate who provided the initial funding to get this project off the ground; the substantial contribution from Angus NHS Trust over the final 18 months which secured the completion of the book; and The Post-Graduate Nutrition & Dietetic Centre, Aberdeen, for their support with production.

The following tables are crown copyright and reproduced with the permission of the Controller of Her Majesty's Stationery Office. Tables 1.1, 1.3, 1.4, 6.1, 12.1 and 12.2, together with Appendix II and Table A1.

Dr Lesley Hyde, Consultant Community Paediatrician, Derby City General NHS Trust, has kindly granted permission for the reproduction of Table 13.5.

Joyce Thompson
Nutrition and Dietetic Manager (Angus NHS Trust)
Stracathro Hospital, Brechin, Angus, DD9 7QA

List of Abbreviations

AA	Arachidonic acid
ADDH	Attention deficit disorder with hyperactivity
ADI	Accepted daily intake
BASCD	British Association for the Study of Community Dentistry
BDA	British Dental Association
BHA	Butylated hydroxyanisole
BHT	Butylated hydroxytoluene
BMA	British Medical Association
BNF	British Nutrition Foundation
CDM	Casein dominant milks
CHD	Coronary heart disease
CMPI	Cow's milk protein intolerance
COMA	Committee on Medical Aspects of Food Policy
DHA	Docosahexanoic acid
DHSS	Department of Health and Social Security
DoH	Department of Health
DRVs	Dietary reference values
EAR	Estimated average requirements
EFAs	Essential fatty acids
EPA	Eicosapentanoic acid
EU	European Union
FMF	Food Manufacturers' Federation
GLA	Gammalinolenic acid
HEA	Health Education Authority
HMSO	Her Majesty's Stationery Office
HPF	Hydrolysed Protein Infant Milk Formula
LBW	Low birth weight
LCPs	Long chain polyunsaturated fatty acids
MAFF	The Ministry of Agriculture, Fisheries and Food
NME sugars	Non-milk extrinsic sugars
OPCS	Office of Population, Censuses and Surveys
RCGP	Royal College of General Practitioners
RCM	Royal College of Midwives
RCP	Royal College of Physicians
RNI	Reference nutrient intake

RTF	Ready to feed
UNICEF	United Nations International Children's Emergency Fund
VLBW	Very low birth weight
WDM	Whey dominant milks
WHO	World Health Organisation

Introduction

This book was developed in response to a request from Angus health visitors for a source of practical information to address the nutritional requirements of children aged 0–5 years. Development took place over two years and the final book is a tribute to the wide range of individuals who were involved throughout the process.

Discussions with health visitors at the start of the project identified the most common nutritional problems they encountered relating to the under fives, and additional information which could usefully be provided for parents and health professionals. Background research for the document included a comprehensive literature search, reference to relevant government reports and consultations with medical, dental and dietetic experts. A document was drafted and circulated to a wide range of health professionals for evaluation and revision.

The book is divided into three sections based on age ranges and each section is subdivided into chapters to provide easy access to this comprehensive practical resource.

Aims

The book aims to enable health professionals to give correct and consistent nutritional advice to parents and carers of the under fives and to identify those children at risk of nutritional inadequacy.

Objectives

The book provides information on:

(1) Nutritional requirements and how these can be met
(2) Areas of specific nutritional concern
(3) How to assess dietary adequacy in respect of energy and iron
(4) Nutritional problems encountered in specific population subgroups
(5) Factors which determine food choices and eating behaviour
(6) Those children who would benefit from referral to a dietitian

Section 1
The First Twelve Months

1. Breastfeeding

> 'Breastfeeding from a woman who is in good health and nutritional status provides a complete food which is unique to the species. There is no better nutrition for healthy infants both at term and during the early months of life.'
>
> Present Day Practice in Infant Feeding, DHSS 1988a.

This chapter covers:

- The advantages of breastfeeding
- Practical dietary advice for breastfeeding mothers
- Factors helpful to breastfeeding

1.1 Composition of human milk

Breast milk provides complete nutrition for an infant and offers immunological and nutritional benefits which cannot be replicated by infant milk formulae. Health professionals have a responsibility to encourage and support breastfeeding.

Colostrum

This is the compositionally distinctive milk which is produced in the first few days after birth. Colostrum has a higher protein content than mature milk and much of the protein is present as immunoglobulins (mainly IgA) which help to protect against infection.

Colostrum has a lower fat content, and therefore lower energy density, than mature milk and is also rich in minerals and vitamins A, D, and B_{12}.

Mature milk

The transition to mature milk is gradual and stimulated by frequent suckling. The composition of mature breast milk is not homogenous, but varies between individuals and during a feed. Given the nature and changing composition of breast milk, calculated compositional values can only represent average approximations. Average composition is given in Table 1.1.

Table 1.1   Composition of human breast milk per 100 ml.

Component	Human milk (mean values)	Component	Human milk (mean values)
Energy (kcal)	70	Protein (g)	1.3
		Lactose (g)	7.0
Vitamin		Fat (g)	4.2
A (µg)	60		
D (µg)	0.01	*Minerals*	
E (mg)	0.35	Sodium (mg)	15
K (µg)	0.21	Potassium (mg)	60
Thiamin (µg)	16	Chloride (mg)	43
Riboflavin (µg)	30	Calcium (mg)	35
Niacin (µg)	620	Phosphorus (mg)	15
B_{12} (µg)	0.01	Magnesium (mg)	3.0
B_6 (µg)	6	Iron (µg)	76
Folate, total (µg)	5.0	Copper (µg)	39
Pantothenic acid	260	Zinc (µg)	295
(µg)		Iodine (µg)	7
Biotin (µg)	0.8		
C (mg)	3.8		

From: The composition of mature human milk (DHSS, 1977).

Recent work has shown the true energy level of breast milk to be significantly less than previously calculated (Lucas *et al.*, 1987).

1.2   Nutritional characteristics of mature milk

Protein
Breast milk has a lower protein concentration than cow's milk and therefore lower renal solute load. The casein:whey protein ratio of breast milk is 40:60 and this produces a soft, digestible curd in the stomach. The whey fraction is compositionally distinct from bovine whey protein and includes antimicrobial proteins such as IgA. The amino acid profile of breast milk is also different from that of cow's milk. Breast milk contains higher levels of cystine, an amino acid important to brain development.

Fat
Fat provides around 50% of the total energy of breast milk. Fat content varies during a feed, being low at the start (**foremilk**), and increasing as the feed progresses (**hindmilk**). The enzyme lipase is present in human milk and enhances a breastfed infant's absorption of

fat. Human milk is rich in **essential fatty acids,** and the long chain polyunsaturated fatty acids required for brain and retinal development (see next section).

Carbohydrate
Carbohydrate is present in the form of lactose. Lactose enhances calcium absorption and helps to create favourable gut flora that protect against gastro-enteritis.

Vitamins
Vitamin levels in breast milk are influenced by a mother's dietary status and are usually sufficient to meet demand. Supplements of vitamins A, C and D for a breastfeeding mother may be required if dietary adequacy is in doubt.

Minerals
Levels of minerals (e.g. iron, zinc) appear to be low in breast milk, but bioavailability is excellent (Woodruff *et al.,* 1977).

1.2.1   Fatty acids and infant milks

Fatty acids are the structural units of most dietary fats including those in breast milk and cow's milk. They are made up of chains of carbon atoms and occur in 'families' or **series.** Most fatty acids can be synthesised in the body, but two of them, **linoleic acid** and **alpha-linolenic acid** cannot. These are described as **'essential' fatty acids** because they must be supplied in the diet.

Linoleic and alpha-linolenic acid are 'parent' fatty acids and can be converted into long chain polyunsaturated fatty acids (LCPs). The LCPs **arachidonic acid** (AA) and **docosahexanoic acid** (DHA) are derived from linoleic acid and alpha-linolenic acid respectively (see Fig. 1.1).

AA and DHA play a crucial part in brain development (Farquharson *et al.,* 1992) and appear to contribute to visual function (Uauy *et al.,* 1992). Adults are able to synthesise AA and DHA but infants, and especially pre-term infants, cannot do so with the same efficiency (Hernell, 1990). Breast milk supplies AA and DHA in 'ready-made' form. Until recently infant milks provided only the 'parent' fatty acids, linoleic and alpha-linolenic acid (see Fig. 1.1). Following studies of pre-term infant feeding and development (Lucas *et al.,* 1989, 1992a) most specialised low birthweight infant milks are now supplemented with

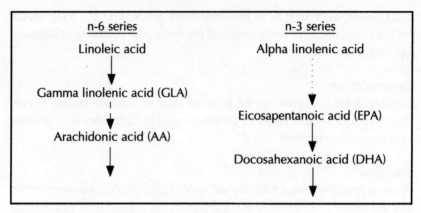

Fig. 1.1 Essential fatty acid metabolism.

AA and DHA. Debate remains as to whether or not standard infant milks should be supplemented and how this should be achieved.

Current evidence makes final conclusions difficult, other than to endorse the superiority of breast milk over commercial products.

1.3 Non-nutritional components of breast milk

1.3.1 Antimicrobial factors

These are summarised in Table 1.2.

1.3.2 Growth factors

Growth factors in breast milk regulate intestinal development.

1.4 Milk production

The physiological aspects of milk production are covered in detail in *Successful Breastfeeding* (RCM, 1991). An understanding of the process is important to provide effective support of breastfeeding.

Milk production can begin only after delivery of the placenta and a decline in placental hormones. The major hormones involved in milk production are **prolactin** and **oxytocin**. The former stimulates milk formation, and the latter stimulates its release. Suckling triggers oxytocin release from the pituitary, and boosts prolactin production which increases milk production. The fact that suckling increases milk production highlights the importance of baby-led feeding.

Table 1.2 Antimicrobial factors in breast milk.

Antimicrobial factors in breast milk	Possible function
Cells Macrophages, e.g. neutrophils Lymphocytes B cells T cells	Engulf bacteria. May transport immunoglobulins. Produce immunoglobulins. Secrete substances which may transfer tuberculin sensitivity to infant.
Immunoglobulin Secretory IgA (mainly) IgG and IgM (present only in small amounts)	Antibodies to a wide range of bacteria, viruses and toxins.
Other factors Lysozyme	Antibacterial enzyme – breaks down bacterial cell walls. The lysozyme content of human milk is 3000 times that of cow's milk.
Lactoferrin	Iron binding protein. Competes with bacteria and yeasts for free iron. Free iron is a microbial growth factor.
Protease inhibitors	Mainly antitrypsin – may reduce digestion of immunoglobulins.
Complement	May assist bacterial cell breakdown.
Vitamin B_{12} and folate binding proteins	Compete with bacteria in gut for vitamin B_{12} and folate. These are microbial growth factors.
Anti-staphylococcal factor	Lipid with anti-staphylococcal action.
Bifidus factor (nitrogen containing polysaccharide)	Promotes growth of beneficial bacteria, and an acidic environment which suppresses pathogens.

Adapted from: Lucas, 1994 and reproduced with permission.

In the first few weeks milk yield is related to high prolactin levels. Once lactation is established, suckling is thought to be a more important factor in maintaining milk production than prolactin levels, since milk remaining in the breast releases a milk production inhibitor.

1.5   Advantages of breastfeeding

The benefits of breastfeeding are well recognised.

- Human milk contains a range of immunoglobulins and other antimicrobial factors (see Table 1.2) which act to block the entry of potential pathogens across the gut mucosa, and reduce risk of infection.
- Breastfeeding for 13 weeks or more has been shown to reduce the incidence of gastro-enteritis and respiratory infections (Howie *et al.*, 1990).
- Breast milk contains optimal ratios of long chain polyunsaturated fatty acids required for brain and retinal development (see Section 1.2.1).
- The solute concentration, and hence potential renal solute load of breast milk, is low.
- The bioavailability of minerals is excellent (Woodruff *et al.*, 1977).
- Breast milk is always available at the right temperature.
- Breast milk is economical for both mother and the National Health Service.
- Breastfeeding has been shown to delay the onset and reduce the severity of allergies in children with a family history of atopic disease (Broadbent & Sampson, 1988).
- Breastfeeding reduces the incidence of necrotising enterocolitis in pre-term babies (Lucas & Cole, 1990).
- There is evidence to suggest that lactation protects against development of breast cancer in premenopausal women (Newcomb *et al.*, 1994).

1.6   Trends in breastfeeding

There has been no significant change in the incidence of breastfeeding, defined as the proportion of infants who were put to the breast, in Europe or the UK since 1980 (see Table 1.3). The Office of Population, Censuses and Surveys (OPCS) survey *Infant Feeding 1990* (White *et al.*, 1992) found that:

Table 1.3 Prevalence of breastfeeding (%) up to 9 months of age in Great Britain and Scotland.

	Great Britain			Scotland		
	1980	**1985**	**1990**	**1980**	**1985**	**1990**
Birth	65	64	63	50	48	50
1 week	57	55	53	44	41	41
6 weeks	41	38	39	32	29	30
4 months	26	26	25	21	22	20

From: White *et al.*, 1992 – Table 2.27.

- 63% of mothers in Great Britain started to breastfeed
- 50% of mothers in Scotland started to breastfeed

Breastfeeding rates vary widely both between and within regions. For example, 81% of mothers in London and south east England chose to breastfeed initially, compared with only 61% of mothers in the north (White *et al.*, 1992). In Scotland, the initial incidence of breastfeeding was found to be highest in the north-east (Orkney, Shetland and Highlands) and lowest in the south-west (Lanarkshire) (Campbell & Jones, 1994).

The 1990 OPCS survey found that the incidence of breastfeeding increased with:

- Mother's social class
- Mother's age
- Age at which mother left full-time education
- Attendance at ante-natal classes
- Positive experience of breastfeeding with previous baby

The influence of friends, knowledge of breastfeeding, and the way mothers themselves were fed as babies were also found to influence the decision to breastfeed. However, the sex of the baby was not a determinant of feeding practice.

1.6.1 Why do mothers stop breastfeeding?

The most common reason for stopping breastfeeding is perceived breast milk insufficiency. Other important reasons in the first two weeks are painful or engorged breasts, baby rejecting breast and no enjoyment when breastfeeding. After two weeks, the main reasons are that the baby is not settling or seems hungry and that breastfeeding takes too long or is tiring.

Having a caesarean delivery under general anaesthetic or a low birthweight infant was also found to be associated with early cessation of breastfeeding. Support and consistent advice from health professionals is a key factor in successful breastfeeding (see also Section 1.5 – Advantages of breastfeeding).

In all cases where problems are encountered:

'Bottle feeding does not resolve breastfeeding problems, but knowledgeable, enthusiastic and sympathetic help can'.

                                                            (RCM, 1991)

How long should a mother breastfeed?

Exclusive breastfeeding for at least four months is recommended by the World Health Organisation and this view is endorsed by UNICEF (WHO/UNICEF, 1989). The Committee on Medical Aspects of Food Policy (COMA) Report *Weaning and the Weaning Diet* (DoH, 1994) states:

'Mothers should be encouraged and supported in breastfeeding for at least four months and may choose to continue to breastfeed as the weaning diet becomes increasingly varied.'

Breast milk supplies all infant nutrient requirements for at least four months and breastfeeding for a minimum of 13 weeks is known to be associated with a reduced incidence of gastrointestinal infection. This protective effect persists beyond the period of breastfeeding and infancy and occurs whether or not solids are given (Forsyth *et al.*, 1993).

As long as appropriate solid foods are introduced by six months of age, a mother should be encouraged to breastfeed as long as she wishes and breastfeeding may continue into the second year.

1.7 Maternal diet

Nutrient needs are detailed in the COMA Report on Dietary Reference Values for Food, Energy and Nutrients for the United Kingdom (DoH, 1991).

1.7.1   Is energy requirement increased during lactation?

Yes, in so far as milk production requires energy expenditure, but metabolic efficiency is thought to be enhanced during lactation, thereby reducing overall energy cost. Energy needs are met by mobilisation of fat stores laid down during pregnancy and energy derived from an increased food intake (see Table 1.4).

Table 1.4   Recommended additional daily (food) energy requirements during lactation.

Stage of lactation	Extra kcals
0–1 month	450
1–2 months	530
2–3 months	570
3–6 months	480
6+ months	240

From: DoH, 1991.

However, individuals show wide variation in post-partum weight loss and hence energy requirements are higher when more than one infant is being fed: However women worldwide lactate successfully on low energy intakes and this may to be due to enhanced metabolic efficiency (Illingworth *et al.*, 1986).

What general advice can I give about increasing energy intake?
In many cases, mother's appetite serves to regulate calorie intake but advice about appropriate food choices may be needed. Foods should be chosen from each of the following food groups daily:

- Milk and dairy foods
- Meat, fish and alternatives
- Bread, other cereals and potatoes
- Fruit and vegetables

Foods in these different groups supply different combinations of nutrients needed for health. (See detailed information in Chapter 6 – Weaning). Dietary **variety** is therefore to be encouraged for all lactating mothers.

Can I give advice on weight loss and dieting?

A low calorie diet may adversely affect the supply and quality of breast milk and intentional 'dieting' should be discouraged until after weaning. Gradual weight loss due to mobilisation of fat stores is not detrimental to milk production. This weight loss, although common during lactation, is not inevitable.

1.7.2   What about fluids?

Fluid requirement is variable between mothers and studies have shown that neither a significant decrease nor a significant increase in maternal fluid intake has any effect on milk production (Dusdieker *et al.*, 1985). Mothers should be advised to drink to satisfy thirst and that dark or strong smelling urine indicates the need to drink more fluids.

1.7.3   What about protein?

An extra 11 g of protein per day is required but this is usually met by an increased food intake.

1.7.4   What about calcium?

Calcium requirements are increased during lactation and a daily intake of 1250 mg is recommended. Approximately 250 mg calcium is provided from:

- 200 ml ($\frac{1}{3}$ pint) whole, semi-skimmed or skimmed milk
- 35g ($1\frac{1}{4}$ oz) cheddar type cheese
- 140g (5 oz) carton of yoghurt

Other sources of calcium are given in Section 13.4.1 – Calcium.

Adolescent mothers are likely to have higher requirements and supplements may be required (Chan *et al.*, 1987). Vegan breastfeeding mothers must maintain an adequate intake of non-dairy calcium-rich foods. (See Chapter 18 – Vegetarian and Ethnic Minority Diets). Supplements may again be required.

1.7.5   What about vitamin D?

Vitamin D is needed for the absorption of calcium from the gut and is essential for effective bone mineralisation. Vitamin D is synthesised through the action of sunlight on skin, but between October and March the necessary ultraviolet-B radiation is not available in Britain

(DoH, 1991). Breast milk contains little vitamin D, especially during winter (Greer *et al.*, 1981). A breastfed infant is largely dependent on good stores at birth and the action of sunlight to maintain vitamin D status. Vitamin D supplementation to achieve an intake of 10 µg per day is recommended for pregnant and lactating women (DoH, 1991). The only useful dietary sources of vitamin D include eggs, 'oily' fish and fortified margarines. Good vitamin D status will:

- Safeguard maternal bone health
- Maximise an infant's vitamin stores at birth
- Maintain vitamin D content of breast milk

Government welfare vitamins are the recommended means of supplementation so as to prevent any risk of toxicity through overdosage (see Section 3.4).

1.7.6 Do breastfed babies require vitamin supplements?

Where maternal vitamin status during pregnancy was good, supplements are not required in the first six months.

From six months, infants consuming breast milk as their main milk should be given supplements and where there is any doubt about maternal vitamin stores, e.g. vegan or Asian mothers, supplementation is recommended from one month (DoH, 1994).

Pre-term infants are at high risk of vitamin depletion and are commonly prescribed supplements prior to hospital discharge. Check local policies.

1.7.7 Iron

Iron requirements are 8.7 mg per day during lactation. This is the same as for a non-lactating woman. It is thought that iron secretion in breast milk may be offset by lactational amenorrhoea (DoH, 1991).

Asian women and those following strict vegetarian or vegan diets should be particularly advised on maintaining high intake of vitamin C, to promote iron absorption from plant sources. Iron absorption is discussed further in Chapter 7.

1.7.8 Dietary exclusion

Maternal diet influences the composition of breast milk but, in general, there is no reason for a breastfeeding mother to exclude any particular food from her diet. Loose stools in the first week after birth relate to the baby's adjustment to milk, and not maternal diet. However, specific food items may cause loose stools in individual babies and a mother may choose to avoid them. Allergens are occasionally transferred in breast milk and can provoke a reaction (Cant *et al.*, 1986); for example, cow's milk in the maternal diet is sometimes found to be associated with eczema in a breastfed baby.

What should I advise if a reaction to cow's milk is suspected?
A trial of milk exclusion from the mother's diet for two weeks can be undertaken. If symptoms improve and then return on reintroduction of cow's milk, referral should be made to a dietitian by a medical practitioner.

Prolonged exclusion of milk without dietetic intervention risks calcium deficiency.

1.7.9 Non nutritive substances

A number of 'non-food' substances are transferred in breast milk. Official guidelines are lacking, but caution is recommended, as shown in Table 1.5.

Table 1.5 'Non-food' substances transferred in breast milk.

Substance	Advice
Alcohol	May cause drowsiness – restrict to an occasional drink.
Caffeine	Is cleared slowly from a baby's system and may cause drowsiness or irritability. Advisable to limit intake of tea, coffee, cola drinks.
Nicotine	Nicotine is expressed in breast milk. Nicotine decreases prolactin levels and smoking can decrease let-down reflex.
Drugs	Should be taken only on medical advice. The British National Formulary (BNF) gives information on drug safety. A hospital information centre will give further advice.
Vitamin preparations	Should be taken only on medical advice.

1.8 Factors found helpful to breastfeeding

Numerous studies have identified factors which are helpful in establishing and maintaining breastfeeding (Salariya *et al.*, 1978; Bloom *et al.*, 1982). Many of these factors are discussed in *Successful Breastfeeding* (RCM, 1991).

1.8.1 Factors helpful to establishment of breastfeeding

- Correct positioning of the baby at the breast to enable successful milk removal and prevent nipple soreness
- Early contact and suckling
- Comfortable feeding posture for mother
- Support and advice at the first feed
- Positive attitude of maternity staff
- Unlimited feeding duration and frequency (de Carvalho *et al.*, 1982)
- Feeding at night
- Unsupplemented breastfeeding, which is also known to influence positively the duration of breastfeeding

1.8.2 Factors helpful to maintaining breastfeeding
(*From:* RCM, 1991; Campbell & Jones, 1994)

- Support of partner
- Level of information received by pregnant women wishing to breastfeed
- Prolonged, intermittent contact with, and support from, health professionals
- Contact with lay breastfeeding groups
- Delayed return to work and less than full-time employment

1.9 Factors found unhelpful to breastfeeding

Anything which interferes with the demand–supply process of lactation, or reduces a mother's confidence in her ability to breastfeed, is detrimental to breastfeeding.

Factors identified as unhelpful to breastfeeding include:

- Delay in putting the baby to the breast
- Rigid feeding schedules
- Additional fluids or feeds (see below)

- Use of infant formula or samples (Bergevin *et al.*, 1983)
- Use of dummies or pacifiers
- Test weighing
- Mother's concern about her milk supply or baby's weight gain
- Negative attitude of father/family
- Conflicting advice from health professionals

Inappropriate hospital practices remain a source of concern in this area (Beeken & Waterston, 1992; Campbell & Jones, 1994). One such example is the use of additional fluids.

Why are additional fluids not recommended?

Giving additional feeds of infant milk or dextrose/glucose to breastfed babies may interfere with milk production and the successful establishment of lactation. This practice is strongly associated with early cessation of breastfeeding (Gray-Donald *et al.*, 1985).

Full term, healthy infants can mobilise stores of glycogen and fat to meet energy requirements after birth. Dextrose/glucose is *not* required to prevent hypoglycaemia and additional fluids have not been found to prevent or resolve physiological jaundice (de Carvalho *et al.*, 1981). Healthy breastfed babies have not been found to require additional fluid in hot weather to prevent dehydration (Goldberg & Adams, 1983).

The practice of giving additional fluids to breastfed babies should be avoided other than in exceptional circumstances.

1.10   Failure to thrive at the breast

Poor weight gain, infrequent wet nappies and an unsettled baby are indicative of underfeeding.

Perceived breast milk insufficiency is the most common reason for mothers stopping breastfeeding (White *et al.*, 1992) but true breast milk insufficiency is rare. Underfeeding is most commonly due to a baby failing to achieve an adequate intake of high calorie hindmilk. This may be due to poor positioning and/or fixing at the breast or an inappropriate feeding time at each breast. Breast engorgement or a mother's tiredness may also affect milk supply.

Breast engorgement/pain → reduced feeding frequency →
reduced milk supply
Mother's tiredness/anxiety/illness → reduced milk supply

These problems require sympathetic management, and detailed advice is to be found in specialist texts such as *Successful Breastfeeding* (RCM, 1991). It should be noted, however, that there are very few mothers who, with sufficient help, are not capable of successful breastfeeding.

Practical management of poor weight gain

(1) Assess baby's wellbeing (urine, bowels, contentment etc.)
(2) Assess degree of growth failure in relation to centile chart, allowing for differences between:
   (a) birth centile – true centile;
   (b) growth patterns of breast and bottle fed babies
(3) Investigate infant's feeding pattern and mother's perception of her milk supply
(4) Ensure correct fixing at the breast
(5) Advise on changed feeding pattern as required
(6) Monitor weight gain closely

Where there is diarrhoea and/or vomiting, an infant failing to thrive must be referred for medical assessment. Continued failure to thrive in the absence of symptoms also requires medical referral (see Section 4.4 – Failure to thrive).

If all attempts to improve lactation fail, a decision has to be made to introduce supplementary feeding with an infant milk. Continuation of some breastfeeding is to be encouraged.

1.11   Changing from breast to bottle feeding

Mothers should understand that the introduction of supplementary feeds will interfere with the cycle of demand and supply, and result in reduced milk production.

Practical points

- A mother wishing to stop breastfeeding should do so gradually
- Combined breastfeeding and formula feeding can be achieved and is a natural progression for an older infant

A first bottle feed should be offered after a shortened breast feed. The feeding bottle may be rejected at first.

- A change of teat shape can be helpful
- For an infant of six months or more, a trainer cup may be used

1.12   Contraindications to breastfeeding

In Great Britain, where infectious diseases are not the primary cause of death during infancy, women who are HIV positive, or those at high risk who have not been serologically tested, should not be advised to breastfeed (DHSS, 1988b; WHO, 1992). The risk of virus transmission from an infected mother to her child has been calculated at 28%, but risk varies with circumstance.

Maternal diabetes, epilepsy and caesarean section are not contra-indications to breastfeeding, but these mothers need additional support and advice. Guidance on other special cases, e.g. cleft palate and Down's Syndrome, is given in *Successful Breastfeeding* (RCM, 1991).

Mothers who are taking certain drugs, e.g. lithium, and babies suffering from the inborn error of metabolism galactosaemia are contraindications to breastfeeding.

1.13   Promotion of breastfeeding

The promotion of breastfeeding can be supported on nutritional, medical and economic grounds.

- Human milk is species specific and ideally suited to infants' nutritional needs.
- Breastfeeding protects against gastrointestinal infection and the development of atopic disease.
- Increasing the number of infants breastfed would reduce hospital admissions for gastrointestinal infections. Since it costs around £300 per day to care for an infant in hospital, potential savings are significant.

Given the evident benefits of improving breastfeeding rates, it is a matter of some concern that the government's advertising budget in support of breastfeeding is around £50 000, whilst that of the infant milk companies is £12 000 000.

It is widely recognised that increasing breastfeeding within the general population is dependent on changing cultural attitudes and this is a long-term process. Considerable scope, however, exists for increasing the prevalence of breastfeeding by increasing the support given to women who choose to breastfeed.

Potential intervention strategies include:

- Extending staff training in breastfeeding management
- Improving information given to mothers wishing to breastfeed
- Tackling current 'unhelpful' practices

These and other strategies are reviewed in an important recent report, *Breastfeeding in Scotland* (Campbell & Jones, 1994).

In conclusion

'Health workers should encourage and protect breastfeeding.'

(WHO/UNICEF (1981)

'All professional staff who are concerned with infant feeding should review their policy and practice to ensure that parents receive adequate advice to encourage the mother to breastfeed her baby.'

DHSS (1988a)

2. Bottle Feeding

> 'Responsible education about bottle feeding does not need to undermine the overriding principle that breastfeeding is superior.'
>
> Present Day Practice in Infant Feeding, DHSS, 1988a

Mothers who choose to bottle feed need information and advice on safe and appropriate feeding.

This chapter covers:

- The differences between breast milk and infant milk
- The differences between types of infant milk
- Advice on the safe preparation of infant milk feeds

2.1 Trends in bottle feeding

The OPCS Survey *Infant Feeding 1990* (White *et al.*, 1992) found that:

- 37% of mothers in Britain bottle fed their babies from birth
- 50% of mothers in Scotland bottle fed their babies from birth
- 75% of all babies in Britain, and 80% of all babies in Scotland, were fully bottle fed at four months of age
- Bottle feeding is becoming increasingly widespread as more mothers supplement breastfeeding with bottle feeds

There is an increased likelihood of bottle feeding with:

- Decreasing social class
- Mother aged under 25
- Mother completing full-time education before the age of 18
- Lack of family history of breastfeeding
- Absence of partner
- Increasing birth order

The reasons most commonly given for planning to bottle feed were:

- Other people can feed the baby
- Mother's previous experience

- Mother does not like of the idea of breastfeeding
- Embarrassment

2.2   Infant milks

Following adoption of *The Infant Formula and Follow-on Formula Regulations 1995* (DoH, 1995), which was implemented in the UK as a response to a European Commission Directive, infant milk formulae are now classified on the basis of their protein content:

- **Infant milk** describes a product where the protein source is entirely derived from cow's milk
- **Infant formula** describes a product where the protein source is not derived from cow's milk, e.g. soya

2.2.1   Composition

The composition of all infant milks complies with the guidelines of the COMA report *Artificial Feeds for the Young Infant* (DHSS, 1980) and the *The Infant Formula and Follow-on Formula Regulations 1995* (DoH, 1995). These 1995 regulations implement the European Commission Directives 91/321/EEC and 92/52/EEC and represent the first mandatory controls on the composition and marketing of breast milk substitutes and follow-on milks.

Infant milks are manufactured from cow's milk which has been modified in the following way:

(1)   Reduction of total protein content, modification of the ratio of insoluble casein to soluble whey protein, adjustment of amino acid profile
(2)   Increase in carbohydrate
(3)   Adjustment of fat composition
(4)   Reduction in mineral content to approximate that of breast milk. Fortification with specific minerals (e.g. iron) and vitamins to compensate for poor bioavailability

Infant milks can be divided into two groups: **whey dominant milks (WDM)** and **casein dominant milks (CDM)**.

In spite of extensive modification, it must be appreciated that infant milk composition can only approximate that of breast milk. Infant milks do not provide the immunological benefits of breast milk (for these see Section 1.3.1) and cannot mimic its changing composition during a feed and throughout lactation.

2.2.2   Whey dominant milk

The composition of whey dominant milk approximates that of breast milk and if breastfeeding is not possible, WDM is generally recommended as the milk of choice from birth.

WDM has:

- Casein:whey protein ratio of 40:60
- Low sodium content
- Low protein content
- Low potential renal solute load

Energy content is based on calculated values for mature breast milk.

A number of the brands shown in Table 2.1 are available in 'ready to feed' (RTF) form.

Table 2.1   Brand names of whey dominant infant milks.

Cow & Gate Premium
Farleys First Milk
Sainsbury's First Menu: First Stage
Milupa Aptamil
SMA Gold
Boots Formula 1

2.2.3   Casein dominant milk

This milk is less highly modified than WDM and has:

- Casein:whey protein ratio of 80:20, similar to that of cow's milk;
- Higher sodium content than WDM and breast milk
- Higher protein content that WDM and breast milk
- Higher potential renal solute load than WDM and breast milk

Energy content is similar to WDM.

A number of the brands shown in Table 2.2 are available in RTF form.

Table 2.2 Brand names of casein
dominant infant milks.

Cow & Gate Plus
Farleys Second Milk
Milupa Milumil
SMA White
Boots Formula 2

2.2.4 Soya infant formulae

These products should not be a first choice breast milk substitute
unless there is specific need to exclude cow's milk products from the
diet. Soya infant formula is considered in Section 8.5 and Section 9.8.5.

2.2.5 Changing milks

The OPCS survey of 1990 found that 41% of mothers bottle feeding at
6–10 weeks had changed the milk they gave their infants. The most
common first change was from a whey dominant milk to a casein
dominant milk. Reasons given for switching milks were:

- Baby not satisfied
- Baby kept being sick
- Constipation

What is the evidence?
Research evidence to support the practice of changing milks is limited.
The type and quantity of casein in milk influences curd formation in
the stomach and delays gastric emptying time (Billeaud *et al.*, 1990).
Infants, however, vary in their gastric emptying time and the satiety
value of casein dominant milk is still questioned (Taitz & Scholey,
1989).

Should changing milks be discouraged?
The practice does not appear to be harmful, but there are good reasons
to discourage changing milks:

(1) The composition of breast milk is ideal for infants' needs. The
    composition of whey dominant infant milk is generally agreed to
    be closer to breast milk than casein dominant milk.
(2) Changing milks when an infant is 'unsettled' does not take

account of other reasons for the apparent failure to settle, e.g. insufficient feeding frequency or feed volume, excessive intake of air or reasons unrelated to feed.

(3) Changing milks can delay diagnosis of underlying disease (Taitz & Wardley, 1990).

(4) Repeated introduction of unfamiliar milks is likely to confuse an infant and create further feeding problems.

Changing milks is considered preferable to the premature introduction of solids.

2.3 Preparation of feeds

All mothers who choose to bottle feed need to be shown how to make up feeds before discharge from the maternity unit, and reinforcement of the procedure may be necessary for some. A high standard of hygiene must be maintained when making up and storing feeds. Bottle fed babies are three times more likely to suffer gastrointestinal infections in their first year (Howie *et al.*, 1990) and water is the main source of microbiological hazard in infant milk feeds (DHSS, 1988a).

All water used for feeds or drinks for infants of less than six months should be boiled and cooled before use (DoH, 1994). Table 2.3 shows the types of water unsuitable for making up feeds.

Feeds must be made the correct strength and in accordance with tin or packet instructions. In the UK dilution is standardised to 1 level scoop of powder to 30 ml cooled, boiled water. Mistakes in making up feeds are common and can risk hypernatraemia and/or excessive weight gain (Taitz & Wardley, 1990).

Example
An extra 2 g infant milk powder at each of eight feeds in a day = 16 g.
16 g infant milk powder = 83 kcal.
At 7 days, 83 kcal > 20% daily energy requirement.
An energy intake persistently greater than requirement risks excessive weight gain.

Feeds should be made up and offered in accordance with manufacturers' instructions. As a general rule:

- Feed on demand
- Use 150 ml/kg body weight as a guideline
- Move gradually from three hourly to four hourly feeds by four months of age

Table 2.3 Types of water not suitable for making up feeds.

Water type	Reason
Softened water	May contain an unacceptably high level of sodium, and risk hypernatraemia (raised serum sodium).
Bottled water* with added minerals	Mineral content of bottled waters is variable. High solute concentrations may lead to overload.
Natural mineral water	Risks fluorosis (Toumba & Curzon, 1994).
Effervescent bottled water	Promotes wind. Variable mineral content.
Filtered water	Microbiologically unsafe: water filters are a breeding ground for bacteria.
Repeatedly boiled water	Contains a high level of sodium.

From: DHSS, 1988a; DoH, 1994.
* The recommended upper limit for sodium in a prepared infant milk feed is 35 mg per 100 ml (DHSS, 1988a), therefore only bottled water with a sodium content of less than 10 mg per 100 ml may be used.

2.4 Microwaves

Microwave ovens should not be used to sterilise feeding bottles without a proper microwave steam sterilising unit.

Microwave ovens should not be used to reheat bottles of milk because:

- Hot milk in the centre of the bottle can cause serious scalding
- Powdered milk proteins can change in microwave conditions

If mothers insist on microwave heating in spite of advice to the contrary:

- Bottles should be inverted several times after heating to ensure equal heat distribution
- The temperature of milk must be tested before feeding

2.5 Infant milk marketing

The Infant Formula and Follow-on Formula Regulations (DoH, 1995) is the first legislation regulating the advertising and promotion of infant milks. Before this came into force infant milk manufacturers generally adhered to a voluntary code of practice drawn up by the (then) Food Manufacturers' Federation (FMF, 1983). This code was based on the International Code of Marketing of Breast Milk Substitutes (WHO/UNICEF, 1981). Whilst the WHO code is endorsed by most industrialised countries' governments, it is not universally implemented (Howard *et al.*, 1993).

Manufacturers of infant milk are recognised as a major source of educational material on infant feeding and there remains a need for independently produced written information (DHSS, 1988a).

Health professionals should be familiar with the articles of the WHO code (WHO/UNICEF 1981) and *The Infant Formula and Follow-on Formula Regulations* (DoH, 1995), and recognise their relevance to professional practice. The main points of the WHO/UNICEF Code on Breast Milk Substitutes are (Smith, 1995):

- Milk formulae should not be advertised to the public
- There must be no free samples issued to the public
- Health workers must not promote these products
- The use of idealised photographs of bottle feeding babies and accompanying health messages, particularly on labels, should cease
- Information to health workers must be factual
- All information on milk substitutes must include reference to the superior nature of breastfeeding and a warning on the costs and potential risks, hazards and disadvantages of substitutes.

3. Problem Solving

> 'A baby's needs seem simple enough in theory...'
>
> Morse, 1988

This chapter covers:

- Advice on the management of infant constipation, posseting and colic
- Supplementary vitamins.

A number of problems are commonly encountered with both breastfed and bottle fed infants which are not due to organic disease. These can often be solved by advice and reassurance.

3.1 Constipation

Constipation may be defined as the infrequent passing of hard stools, i.e. every 5–7 days or so.

Constipation is very rare in breastfed infants since breast milk tends to have a mild laxative effect. It is more common in infants fed infant milks, but babies' bowel habits do vary considerably and parents' expectations of what constitutes a 'normal' habit may be unrealistic. Constipation in infants is usually due to an inadequate fluid intake. This may be the result of over-concentrated feeds.

Management of constipation

Breastfed baby

- Obtain accurate report of stool frequency and consistency
- Establish mother's perception of a normal bowel habit
- Investigate baby's feeding pattern
- Ensure mother is taking a varied diet and adequate fluids

Bottle fed baby

- Investigate feeding pattern and bowel habits as for breastfed baby

- Check total fluid intake and concentration of feeds
- Encourage additional drinks of cooled, boiled water between feeds
- Babies over six weeks can be offered very dilute unsweetened fruit juice (e.g. one teaspoon unsweetened fruit juice or baby fruit juice in 50 ml cooled, boiled water)
- For a baby over three months, this can be increased to 2–3 teaspoons unsweetened fruit juice in 50 ml cooled, boiled water
- Sugar should not be added to the feeding bottle. This exerts an osmotic effect and will further reduce a baby's fluid stores, with the potential risk of dehydration and dental caries

Weaned baby

- Consider diet, fluid intake and bowel habits
- Gradually increase fibre intake
- Encourage extra fruit and vegetable purées, especially pulses, i.e. beans, peas and lentils
- Infants over six months can be given small quantities of unrefined cereal products, e.g. wholemeal bread, porridge
- Give extra fluid as water or well diluted unsweetened fruit juice

Bran is the dry, flaky substance made from the outer layers of wheat which are removed during the manufacture of white flour.

Unprocessed bran should *never* be given to infants or young children as it reduces the absorption of some micronutrients. Severe, persistent constipation requires medical management.

3.2 Posseting (gastro-oesophageal reflux)

Posseting is usually due to a muscle weakness at the point where the oesophagus joins the stomach. It is not a definitive feature of food allergy or intolerance. Posseting generally decreases with time, especially once solids are introduced. In a small number of cases it may be due to hiatus hernia.

Posseting requires medical investigation if there is:

- Poor weight gain
- Regurgitation of blood
- Respiratory symptoms

Management of posseting

- Check milk intake. Overfeeding can cause posseting.
- Check feeding technique. Posseting is exacerbated by swallowing air.
- Encourage upright positioning after feeds.
- Thickening feeds assists the retention of milk. This is usually carried out under dietetic supervision. Commonly used prescribable products include Vitaquick* (Vitaflo), Instant Carobel (Cow and Gate) and Nestargel (Nestlé).
- Breastfed babies can be offered feed thickeners as a paste on a spoon prior to a feed.
- Changing milks will not resolve posseting.

* *Not* prescribable for infants under one year except in cases of failure to thrive.

3.3 Colic

'Severe pain resulting from periodic spasm in an abdominal organ'

(Roper, 1980)

Colic is characterised by vigorous, periodic crying episodes and drawing up the legs, indicative of abdominal pain. It is common in both bottle fed and breastfed babies, usually occurring between six weeks and three months of age and often in the evening.

In some breastfed babies colic may be associated with an inadequate intake of hindmilk, causing rapid gastric emptying and lactose over-load (Wooldridge & Fisher, 1988), but in many cases the cause is unknown.

Is colic associated with food intolerance?
A joint report of the 1984 Royal College of Physicians and British Nutrition Foundation (RCP/BNF, 1984) concluded that the association between infantile colic and food intolerance was unproven and subsequent studies have failed to provide conclusive proof.

Colic should not be used as a reason for stopping breastfeeding or changing infant milks. Withdrawal of cow's milk from the diet of breastfeeding mothers may be successful in a small number of cases, but the evidence in support of this practice is tenuous.

Exclusion of milk and milk products from a breastfeeding mother's diet requires dietetic supervision.

Management of colic

- Check and advise a change in feeding pattern where appropriate.
- Gripe water preparations are now alcohol-free and may be given to babies over one month. Active ingredients include sodium bicarbonate and/or activated dimethicone, which act to relieve flatulence.
- Colic drops may be used, e.g. Infacol (contain dimethicone).
- Herbal drinks should not be given to settle babies who are suffering from colic unless they are verified as sugar free. Some brands contain dextrose which is highly cariogenic when fed from a bottle.
- Gentle movement seems to settle some babies.
- Reassure parents that, in the absence of other symptoms, colic is not a cause of medical concern and will eventually resolve.

3.4   Vitamins

Vitamin supplements for mothers and young children were introduced as part of the Welfare Foods Scheme in the 1940s. Pregnant mothers, breastfeeding mothers and children under five years of age in families receiving Income Support qualify for free vitamins (see Appendix III).

A daily dose of five Department of Health vitamin drops supplies:

- Vitamin A (retinol equivalents) – 200 µg
- Vitamin C – 20 mg
- Vitamin D_3 – 7 µg

Until recently vitamin supplementation was recommended for all children aged six months up to at least two years (DHSS, 1988a). In practice, the Ministry of Agriculture, Fisheries and Food (MAFF) Survey *Food and Nutrient Intake of British Infants aged 6–12 months* (Mills & Tyler, 1992) found less than half of infants surveyed received vitamin supplements. Whilst dietary intakes of vitamin A and C appeared adequate, intake of vitamin D was only 50% of that recommended without supplements. Vitamin D intakes were lowest in infants aged 9–12 months.

Current recommendations
The 1994 COMA report *Weaning and the Weaning Diet* recognises that bottle fed infants consuming more than 500 ml of vitamin fortified infant milk per day, do not require additional supplements.

Vitamin supplements are recommended for:

- Infants over six months of age, having breast milk as their main milk
- Breastfed infants over one month where maternal vitamin status is in doubt (see Section 1.7.6)
- Bottle fed infants consuming less than 500 ml infant milk per day
- 'At risk infants' over one month of age (see below)
- All children from 1–5 years, unless dietary adequacy can be assured

Infants '**at risk**' of vitamin deficiency include pre-term infants, Asian infants, and those on restrictive diets, e.g. vegan. Risk of vitamin D deficiency in particular is increased between the ages of six months and three years because of the rate at which calcium is laid down in bone (DoH, 1991).

Is there risk of vitamin overdose?

There is no risk when Department of Health vitamins are given at the recommended dosage of five drops in conjunction with:

- Infant milk or follow-on milk
- Breast milk
- Weaning diet

Vitamin and mineral supplements other than the above should not be given without medical recommendation because there is danger of overdose with these (see Section 17.3 – Supplementary government vitamins).

4. Growth

> 'Growth is one of the most sensitive indicators of health in childhood.'
>
> Hindmarsh & Brook, 1986

This chapter covers:

- The importance of effective growth monitoring
- The concept of 'failure to thrive'
- Infants who require medical assessment due to poor growth

Poor growth may be indicative of underlying disease, poor nutrition, emotional neglect or a combination of these factors. Growth therefore requires regular and effective monitoring throughout infancy and childhood.

4.1 Importance of good growth in infancy

It is difficult to underestimate the significance of good growth in the first year. Poor weight gain and slowed growth in infancy are associated with developmental delay, increased risk of ischaemic heart disease and increased risk of diabetes in adult life.

In infancy, growth is strongly related to nutritional adequacy. Measurement of growth therefore measures nutritional adequacy.

4.2 Growth monitoring

Early detection of growth failure depends on effective monitoring. This requires:

- Regular measurements
- Accurate measurements
- Accurate transcription of data to centile chart
- Appropriate action on results

What measurements should be made?
Weight and length/height require routine measurement and assess-

ment. Head circumference may be useful in children under two years of age. Measurement of height and/or weight velocity may be made when growth adequacy is in doubt. A single measurement of each parent (where possible) is recommended to enable calculation of an infant's adult height potential.

How often should measurements be made?
There is no nationally followed standard of measurement intervals. A minimum for weight monitoring in infancy is suggested as birth, the six week check and times of immunisation (Edwards *et al.*, 1990). Three monthly measurements of all indicators have also been proposed.

How can errors be limited?
Attention to detail is important. The following checklist can be used to limit measurement errors:

(1) Measurement by same observer/s wherever possible
(2) Measurement procedure standardised
(3) Appropriate and regularly calibrated measuring instrument
(4) Measurement made at same time of day
(5) Subject in same state of undress
(6) Subject positioned correctly

4.2.1 Growth charts

Growth charts based on centile distribution curves allow comparison of an infant's growth with that of an age-matched reference population. Commonly used curves are those of Tanner *et al.* (1966). These curves have been misused in a study however (Freeman *et al.*, 1995) because accurate monitoring of children below the third centile was difficult and the original curves did not reflect the growth patterns of children in the 1990s (children are now taller and bigger). Growth charts based on the revised curves allow clearer identification of children at risk of growth failure and encourage calculation of adult height potential. (See Resource List at the back of the book: Child Growth Foundation and Castlemead Publications.)

When using growth (centile) charts remember:

• Record measurements as a single point to prevent ambiguity
• For infants born before 37 weeks, plot measurements from week of birth for at least 12 months

- Growth along lower centiles is not in itself an indication of 'failure to thrive' (FTT) (see Section 4.4). However, weight and height should not differ by more than two major centiles

4.3   Specific measurements

4.3.1   Weight

Measurement of weight is a straightforward and reasonably accurate measure of growth. A weight loss of up to 10% of an infant's birth weight is to be expected by day three, but this can be greater in pre-term infants.

Expected weight gain for a healthy, term infant is:

- 200 g per week in the first three months
- 150 g per week in the second three months
- 100 g per week in the third three months
- 50–75 g per week in the fourth three months
- 2.5 kg during the second year

In general, birth weight doubles in the first 5–6 months and trebles during the first year. Birth weight, however, is a poor indicator of an infant's 'true' centile position since birth weight is largely determined by maternal and not genetic influences. Weight at 4-8 weeks shows better correlation with centile position at 12 months (Edwards *et al.*, 1990). This should be taken into account when monitoring weight.

4.3.2   Linear growth

Length reflects bone growth and is therefore a better indicator of long-term growth and nutritional adequacy than weight. Expected linear growth is:

- 25 cm in length during the first year
- 12 cm in length during the second year

Accurate assessment of linear growth is difficult in young children and should be carried out by skilled practitioners.

Remember:
Measure supine length until about two years of age, and height thereafter. These two values are likely to be different. When changing

from length to height measurement, one recording of both length and height should be made to allow fair comparison of subsequent height measurements.

4.3.3 Head circumference

Expected rate of growth is:

- 1 cm per month in the first year
- 2 cm in all of the second year

This reflects rapid brain growth in the first year. Accurate measurement depends on:

- Use of non-stretching tape measure
- Passing tape around forehead, eyebrows and occiput
- Making two measurements

4.3.4 Growth velocity

Growth velocity (rate of growth) is rarely part of routine monitoring, but two observations relating to rate of growth are significant:

(1) Breastfed babies show a different pattern of growth from bottle fed babies
(2) Growth rate in childhood is not constant. Slowed growth is therefore not always indicative of growth failure

4.4 Failure to thrive

What is 'failure to thrive'?
Failure to thrive (FTT) is not a specific disease, but rather an observation of poor growth. It has been described as when 'the rate of growth fails to meet the potential expected of a child of that age' (Frankl & Zeisel, 1988). Children with mild FTT may appear to be well, and growth screening is therefore central to early detection. Prolonged FTT must be prevented since it is associated with long-term linear growth retardation and developmental delay.

4.4.1 Identifying failure to thrive

FTT should not be considered as growth 'below' any given centile, because some infants are constitutionally small. For example, infants of very low birth weight or of short parents are more likely to be of short stature (Kitchen *et al.*, 1989). Falling from a predicted growth centile is an important indicator of possible FTT, especially where more than one centile has been crossed. Some deviation from the weight centile in the first six months is not uncommon however. Just as light for date infants may show early 'catch up' growth, other infants may show a period of slow growth and 'catch down' weight (Marcovitch, 1994). The implications of this are uncertain. Careful monitoring of weight and lengths is required.

What should I do about an infant 'falling off' a centile?
Where there is deviation from the weight centile:

- Check length/height centile position
- Monitor and follow up if there is no deviation from length centile and infant appears healthy

Refer for medical assessment:

- If there is deviation from the height centile
- If infant appears ill or lethargic
- If downward trend in weight centile position continues
- If weight and height differ from each other by more than two major centiles
- If there is any doubt about wellbeing

4.4.2 Causes of failure to thrive

Distinction has been made between **organic** and **non-organic** FTT. This is now thought to be inappropriate since undernutrition is the primary cause of growth failure in all cases of non-organic FTT and also in the majority of organic cases (Skuse, 1992). In medical conditions, FTT may be due to malabsorption, or inadequate intake or increased requirements.

Malabsorption

- Cystic fibrosis
- Coeliac disease
- Cow's milk protein intolerance
- Lactose intolerance
- Acute gastrointestinal infection

Inadequate intake or increased requirements

- Chronic illness, e.g. asthma
- Post-operative needs
- Impaired ability to feed (mental/physical)
- Acute infection

Where FTT is of non-medical origins, poor energy intake may be due to:

- Breast-feeding failure
- Inappropriate weaning diet
- Inappropriate dietary restriction
- Food refusal

The causes of non-organic FTT are often complex and almost always multifactorial. Social, psychological, financial or a combination of factors may be involved as illustrated by the following examples.

- Lack of support for mother → fatigue + anxiety → stressful meal times → infant food refusal → failure to thrive
- Lack of money + poor cooking skills → inappropriate weaning diet → failure to thrive
- Overawareness of 'Healthy eating' → inappropriate low fat diet → poor energy intake → failure to thrive

All cases of failure to thrive need detailed, individual assessment and medical referral should be made if there is any doubt about wellbeing.

5. Pre-term and Low Birth Weight Infants

'Infants born pre-term are nutritionally vulnerable.'

Weaning and the Weaning Diet, DoH, 1994

This chapter covers:

- The reasons why low birth weight infants are at risk of nutritional inadequacy
- Sources of specialist advice
- When a low birth weight infant can start weaning

Pre-term and other low birth weight infants require specialist care. They are a group at high nutritional risk and needs must be assessed on an individual basis. The following is an overview of nutrition knowledge in this area, and generalised management in the community. Care of individual infants should be based on the advice of the special care unit of discharge and a dietitian.

5.1 Classification

- Normal (term) birth weight   = 3.3 – 3.5 kg
- Low birth weight (LBW)   = < 2.5 kg
- Very low birth weight (VLBW) = <1.5 kg

Pre-term infants are those born before 37 weeks gestation. Prematurity is one cause of low birth weight; two thirds of LBW infants are born pre-term and have a size appropriate for gestational age. Approximately one third of LBW infants show interuterine growth retardation and are 'small for date'. The nutritional requirements and clinical management of these two groups are not identical.

5.2 Nutrient needs

Requirements have to be defined and met on an individual basis, but all low birth weight infants are considered to be 'at risk' of nutritional inadequacy.

Pre-term infants have:

- Low nutrient stores, e.g. calcium, zinc, iron
- Immature organ and enzyme systems
- High nutrient requirements

Small for date infants have lower energy stores (fat and glycogen) than normal birth weight infants, and are prone to hypocalcaemia. Nutrient requirements are high. In practical terms, small infants risk inadequate bone mineralisation, vitamin and mineral deficiencies, and prolonged sub-optimal growth.

The ideal growth rate and nutrient requirements of low birth weight infants are not known. Since nutrient deprivation in early life is thought to exert a significant effect on long-term outcome (Lucas *et al.*, 1989), optimum nutrition is required from birth. It is no less important that good nutrition is maintained throughout the first year. Low weight at one year shows strong correlation with increased risk of diabetes and coronary heart disease in later life (Barker *et al.*, 1989; Hales *et al.*, 1991).

LBW infants start from a position of nutritional disadvantage. Achieving good catch-up growth is dependent on optimum nutrition. Current knowledge on the nutrient requirements of LBW infants is summarised in a number of reviews (ESPGAN, 1987; Neu *et al.*, 1990).

5.3 Early feeding of LBW infants

Nutrient needs are determined on an individual basis, and feeding methods and regimens vary considerably. Milks used to feed pre-term infants are:

- Mother's breast milk
- Mother's nutrient supplemented breast milk
- Banked breast milk
- Specialised 'low birth weight' infant milk
- Standard infant milks

The use of a combination of different milks is common.

5.3.1 Pre-term breast milk

Mother's breast milk is known to confer immunological protection, reduce the risk of necrotising enterocolitis (Lucas & Cole, 1990), contribute to gut maturation and enhance neurological development.

Breast milk alone, however, may not always be nutritionally adequate to support optimum pre-term, post natal growth.

5.3.2 'Low birth weight' infant milks

Low birth weight milks have a higher nutrient density than standard infant milks. They are for use in hospital only, usually until a weight of about 2 kg is achieved. The majority of low birth weight milks are fortified with long chain polyunsaturated fatty acids (LCPs) because the capacity of a pre-term infant's ability to synthesise these is limited (see Section 1.2.1). Nutrient enriched infant milks are available for pre-term infants after discharge into the community (see Section 5.4.1). These are different from low birth weight milks.

5.4   Management of LBW infants in the community

Pre-term infants are often discharged at a weight of around 2 kg, significantly less than that of a healthy, term infant, and unless good catch-up is achieved growth can remain retarded at 18 months. Since many aspects of a pre-term infant's care may continue to be determined by a hospital team, the following should only be considered as general information.

5.4.1   Energy requirements

It is highly desirable that all LBW infants achieve good growth and catch-up growth in the first year (see Section 5.2). The diet after hospital discharge must therefore provide adequate energy to enable this to occur. At a weight of 2 kg or more it has been customary to give pre-term infants unsupplemented breast milk or a standard infant milk. However, if infant milk is given, there is evidence to suggest that nutrient enriched infant milks may be more suited to pre-term infant nutrient needs than standardised infant milks and may facilitate better growth and bone mineralisation (Lucas *et al.*, 1992b). The composition of nutrient enriched infant milks is somewhere between that of low birth weight milks used in hospitals and standard infant milks.

Two enriched milks are currently available but are neither prescribable nor available on the welfare food scheme: Farley's Premcare and Cow & Gate Nutriprem 2.

Advice should be sought from a paediatric specialist about the use of these milks.

5.4.2 Vitamins and minerals

Different combinations of supplementary vitamins and minerals will be required by individual infants. This should be determined before hospital discharge; most hospitals will have their own policies. Pre-term infants have reduced iron stores, and supplements may be prescribed from 6–8 weeks until the end of the first year. Excessive iron intake is associated with increased risk of infection and supplements may not always be appropriate if iron supplemented formula is taken in large amounts. Again, this will be determined on an individual basis.

5.4.3 Growth

Following discharge, LBW infants may well consume surprisingly large volumes of milk, e.g. 250 ml/kg/day is not unusual. Provided the infant tolerates this amount, i.e. is not vomiting, there will be no cause for concern and catch-up growth will be good.

LBW infants require careful monitoring to ensure satisfactory growth is maintained. Weight and length should be measured regularly. Reduced linear growth can be associated with an inadequate supply of bone minerals (calcium, phosphorus).

LBW infants showing either poor weight gain or reduced linear growth should always be referred for immediate assessment.

How should LBW measurements be plotted on centile charts?
The 1994 Child Growth Standards specify:

- For an infant born before 37 completed weeks, measurements should be plotted from the week of birth for at least 12 months
- For later deliveries, measurements can be plotted from expected date of delivery

5.4.4 Weaning

There is no 'ideal' age at which weaning should commence, but weaning is not recommended before 16 weeks post-delivery, or before an infant is 5 kg in weight (Lawson, 1991). Pre-term babies may never be able to take 'full bottles', i.e. over 180 ml each feed, and this is therefore not an appropriate consideration for starting weaning. Babies with persistent chronic lung disease, or those who have experienced long periods of non-oral feeding, e.g. total parenteral feeding or nasogastric feeding, are at particular risk of developing feeding problems and weaning difficulties. A speech and language therapist may be able to offer valuable assistance in these situations. The degree of prematurity and developmental level need to be taken into account; weaning is inappropriate until an infant has lost the extrusion reflex. The midpoint between 16 weeks chronological age and 16 weeks corrected age may be used as a guide as to when to start (Lawson, 1991).

Example

When could an infant who is 6 weeks pre-term start solids?

For an infant 6 weeks pre-term, 16 weeks corrected age
$$= 22 \text{ weeks chronological age}$$
Midpoint of two ages $= (16 + 22) \div 2$
$$= 19 \text{ weeks chronological age}$$

Weaning could start at 19 weeks provided weight is 5 kg

Practical points (see also Chapter 6 – Weaning)

- First foods should be bland, of a thin, smooth consistency and of low allergenicity, e.g. baby rice, fruit purée.
- As weaning progresses, care must be taken to ensure energy dense foods are given. Large quantities of fruit and vegetables are of low energy density and not appropriate.
- Examples of energy dense weaning foods are cereals mixed with milk, meat/chicken purées (see Table 5.1).
- Delaying the introduction of foods associated with allergic reaction e.g. cow's milk, wheat, eggs (see Section 9.3) until 6 months of age is

Table 5.1 Energy content of weaning foods.

Food	kcal/100 g
Carrot purée	20
Unsweetened fruit purée	50
Baby rice mixed with breast or infant milk	90
Jar/can savoury baby food	60–80
Minced meat ($\frac{1}{3}$) and potato ($\frac{2}{3}$)	150

From: Thomas, 1994 (Reproduced with permission.)

recommended if there is a family history of atopic disease. This should be discussed with a dietitian.

- Weaning foods can be fortified with special energy supplements if weight gain is poor. Any infant showing poor weight gain should be referred to a dietitian so that this can be considered.

6. Weaning

> 'Weaning is the process of expanding the diet to include food and drinks other than breast milk or infant formula.'
>
> Weaning and the Weaning Diet, DoH, 1994

This chapter covers:

- Nutritional and developmental reasons for weaning
- Advice on suitable weaning foods for different ages
- Advice on the preparation of home-made foods
- Food groups and the importance of dietary variety

6.1 Introduction

Weaning is a time of nutritional vulnerability. It represents a period of dietary transition just when nutritional requirements for growth and brain development are high. A nutritionally adequate weaning diet is essential for achieving optimum growth in the first year. Growth in the first year influences both the wellbeing of the child and the long-term health of the adult. Advice about good weaning practice is needed by many mothers. It can otherwise be a time of considerable confusion when detrimental dietary habits may be established.

6.2 Reasons for weaning

There are important nutritional and developmental reasons for introducing solid food.

Nutritional

- After about six months of age, breast milk or infant milk alone cannot meet an infant's energy requirements
- Birth stores of iron and zinc are likely to be depleted by six months. These minerals must then be supplied in the diet

Developmental

- Introduction of different tastes and textures promotes biting and chewing skills
- Chewing improves the mouth and tongue co-ordination which is important for speech development
- Failure to introduce different textures and tastes by 6–7 months can result in their rejection later (Illingworth, 1964)

6.3 Age of weaning

Weaning is a gradual process which does not start at a given age or weight. Current guidelines state:

'The majority of infants should not be given solid foods before the age of four months, and a mixed diet should be offered by the age of six months'

(DoH, 1994)

In practice, the 1990 OPCS study (White *et al.*, 1992) found that 68% of infants in the UK had been given some solid food by three months of age and a further survey that year (Mills & Tyler, 1992) found that 52% of infants aged three months had been given solid food.

Why do mothers start weaning so early?

A number of factors are thought to be involved. These include:

- Baby perceived to be 'unsettled'
- Desire to have baby sleep all night
- Desire to see baby progressing to 'next stage'
- Peer group pressure
- Family advice

The 1990 OPCS survey found early weaning to be more common when a baby is bottle fed, is of a lower socio-economic group or has a mother who smokes.

Is early weaning harmful?

This is a controversial area and evidence is conflicting. The risk of adverse effects depends on many factors, including whether an infant is breast or bottle fed, family history of atopic disease and the age of early weaning. There are, however, good reasons for delaying weaning.

6.3.1   Reasons to delay weaning

Developmental

- Young infants have poor head control and cannot maintain a position for swallowing unaided.
- An infant's extrusion ('spitting out') reflex persists for several months after birth.
- The ability to move food about the mouth and chew does not develop readily before 3–4 months.
- Young infants are reluctant to experiment with new tastes and textures. Rejection of food is common and may prevent later dietary diversity.
- The temptation to add solid food to a feeding bottle is greater. This practice risks both choking and promotion of dental caries.

Physiological

- Renal function is limited at birth, and takes time to mature. The increased renal solute load of solid food can increase risk of dehydration.
- Gut enzyme efficiency takes several months to develop. Early solids may be poorly digested (Milla, 1988).
- Giving solids before 12 weeks has been associated with an increased risk of respiratory disease (Forsyth *et al.*, 1993).
- Early weaning has been associated with an increased incidence of eczema (Fergusson *et al.*, 1990), particularly in families prone to allergy.

Nutritional

- Milk alone can supply all of an infant's nutrient requirements until about 4–6 months of age.
- Solids, given close to a breast feed, can reduce the absorption of nutrients (e.g. iron) from the milk.

What can be done about early weaning?
The situation can often be anticipated and therefore possibly averted. Discuss weaning and suitable first solids as early as possible (before two months) and involve all interested parties (e.g. Granny). It may be helpful to highlight all relevant, negative aspects of early weaning,

including the mess. Setting a target starting date gives something to plan towards.

For the 'unsettled' baby

- Check weight gain and reassure if adequate.
- Breastfeeding?
  Examine breastfeeding practices:
  (1) Frequency
  (2) Length of time at breast
  (3) Positioning
- Bottle feeding?
  (1) Check dilution of feeds
  (2) Increase feed frequency
  (3) Try drinks of cooled, boiled water between feeds
- Stress that giving solids does not guarantee a good night's sleep
- As a last resort, suggest changing to a casein dominant milk

What about an infant who has started solids before four months?

- Ensure intake of breast milk or infant milk is sufficient to meet energy needs for growth
- Check solids are not added to a feeding bottle
- Advise government supplementary vitamins if there is any doubt about milk intake or a breastfeeding mother's vitamin status
- Advise suitable low allergenic 'first foods'
- Monitor variety and adequacy of the weaning diet

6.4   Practical points about weaning

- A mother's attitude is important. Encourage a relaxed approach; a peaceful atmosphere is required and television or family noise are rarely helpful.
- Safety should be emphasised from the start. Because of the risk of choking, infants must never be left alone. If choking occurs:
  (1) Place the infant face down along forearm or lap
  (2) The head should be supported, but tipped below chest
  (3) Tap firmly between shoulders
- Tiredness or hunger may frustrate the process, so suggest offering first foods halfway through a daytime feed when this is less likely to be a problem.
- Weaning is messy and mothers need to be prepared for this.

- Utensils should be appropriate. A shallow plastic spoon which allows a baby to suck food is recommended at first.
- Food should not be forced on a baby. A baby ready for solid food will take it. Weaning is a learning process for a baby and therefore takes time.
- The process of reducing milk feeds should be gradual and determined by the amount of solids taken, growth and the infant's contentment.
- Initially drop one milk feed during the day, e.g. lunch time, once the infant is well established on solids, i.e. consuming a main course at around 6–7 months.
- By eight months a second milk feed may be dropped, e.g. mid-afternoon or mid-morning.

6.5   The first stage: 4–6 months

Suitable first weaning foods include vegetable and fruit purées, non-wheat cereals, unsweetened yoghurt. The quantity, consistency, flavour, potential allergenicity and preparation of first foods all need to be considered.

6.5.1   Quantity

Only tiny quantities are required initially. One teaspoon is often enough, although some babies may take two or three. The small quantity of food consumed in the first stage of weaning is of little nutritional value. Breast or infant milk will remain the major source of nutrients until a fully mixed diet is achieved. The aim is to accustom an infant to taking food from a spoon. Increasing the quantity of solid food given and the frequency with which it is offered depend on an infant's willingness to take it, but solid food should be accepted two to three times per day by about six months of age.

6.5.2   Consistency

First foods need to be of a thin, smooth purée consistency to allow a baby to use the sucking reflex. First foods can readily be made at home, but parents may need advice about how to purée foods, as shown in Table 6.1.

Home-made purées should be thickened gradually as a baby develops the ability to move food to the back of the mouth. 'Wet' manufactured infant foods in jars and tins offer the convenience of ready-

Table 6.1 Making purées.

Utensil	Comments
Fork	Foods need to be very soft, e.g. banana, ripe pear.
Grater	The fine section of grater is good for 'mushing' fruit, cooked carrot etc.
Sieve/tea strainer	More practical initially. Fine mesh needed. Not all foods will sieve effectively.
Hand held blender	Good for small quantities, but texture not always even.
Food mill	Useful, affordable.
Liquidiser	Not good for small quantities.
Food processor	Impractical for small quantities unless mill attachment used.

made purées; dried baby foods require mixing to purée consistency in accordance with packet instructions.

6.5.3 Salt and sugar

Salt should not be added to weaning foods.

- Increasing salt intake increases renal solute load. A baby's renal function takes several months to reach normal efficiency and a high renal solute load increases water lost in the urine. This can, in certain circumstances, lead to hypernatraemia and the risk of dehydration.
- Adding salt may encourage a preference for salty foods; most under fives show an increased liking for salty foods as they get older. In the long term, this may have an adverse effect on blood pressure.

Use sugar sparingly.

- Adding sugar appears to encourage a preference for sweet foods.
- A high intake of sugars is associated with a high risk of dental decay (see Chapter 10 – Dental Health).
- A preference for sweet foods may lead to rejection of nutritious savoury foods later.

- A preference for sweet foods can contribute to excessive weight gain.
- Small amounts of sugar may be added to sour fruits to increase palatability, e.g. apples or rhubarb.
- Unsweetened cereals and yoghurts should be encouraged.

6.5.4 Flavour

First weaning foods should be bland and smooth, but once food is accepted from a spoon, introduction to a variety of different tastes should be encouraged. The period from 4–6 months is thought to be one when infants will accept any new taste, and familiarisation at this age prevents food rejection later (Skuse, 1993). Introduction of new foods one at a time is only considered advisable where there is a strong family history of allergy (DoH, 1994), but the gradual introduction of new foods may facilitate taste differentiation.

6.5.5 Gluten

Gluten is a protein found in wheat, rye, oats and barley. Coeliac disease is an intolerance to gluten associated with intestinal damage and nutrient malabsorption. It is known to run in families and the exact mechanism of the intolerance is unknown. In the past coeliac disease has often been diagnosed during weaning, following the introduction of gluten-containing foods. The decline in the incidence of infants with coeliac disease may, in part, be due to a reduction of gluten in early weaning foods.

For the majority of infants, gluten-containing foods present little hazard, but 'at risk' infants cannot always be identified in advance. Current guidelines therefore recommend that cereals given to infants of less than six months should preferably be gluten-free (DoH, 1994). Where there is a family history of coeliac disease, further delay in the introduction of gluten-containing foods may be considered appropriate. Advice should be sought from a dietitian.

The following foods contain gluten, and are therefore not generally advised before six months:

- Most rusks, whole or granulated (one gluten-free brand is available)
- Wheat-based cereals, e.g. Weetabix
- Oats/oat cereals
- Multi-grain cereals

- Some varieties of dried infant meals or desserts
- Bread, all varieties

It is unclear whether delaying the introduction of gluten prevents coeliac disease or simply delays the clinical presentation of the disease, but since the older child is nutritionally less vulnerable than the infant, delay in presentation is highly beneficial.

6.5.6 Allergenicity

Food allergy is discussed fully in Chapter 9 – Food Intolerance and Allergy. Infants are most vulnerable to the initiation of food allergy in the first months of life and the risk of allergy is greatly increased by family history of atopic disease such as eczema and asthma. For these 'at risk' infants, potential food allergens should be avoided until at least six months of age.

Common food allergens include:

- Cow's milk
- Eggs
- Citrus fruits
- Nuts
- Wheat
- Fish

6.5.7 Are home-made or commercial baby foods better?

Both have a place. The use of appropriately prepared home-made foods should be encouraged, but recent research shows that they are not always nutritionally sound (Morgan *et al.*, 1993; Stordy *et al.*, 1993). Commercial products are convenient and their content conforms to strict compositional guidelines. Quantities of food eaten are tiny at first so preparation must be straightforward and practical.

Home-made foods

- Encourage familiarity with common foods
- Encourage early integration into the family diet
- Prevent overdependence on commercial products
- Can be cheaper
- Should be made following the advice below

Manufactured foods

- Provide convenience
- Allow economical use of small quantities
- Have a regulated composition
- May be fortified with specific nutrients, e.g. vitamin C, iron

Advice

When home-made or manufactured foods are used, food safety principles should be discussed in relation to their preparation (see Chapter 11). Advice should include:

- Storage of foods (and left-overs)
- Reheating
- Use of microwave
- Avoidance of adding salt and sugar
- Foods to avoid

Guide to first stage foods

✓ = suitable   ✖ = unsuitable   **P** = preparation

Fruit	
✓	Fresh pear, banana, peach, apricot, melon; stewed apple, pear, apricot; tinned fruit in unsweetened juice, e.g. pear, peach.
✖	Citrus fruits, fruits with seeds (e.g. raspberry).
P	Wash and peel fresh, ripe, unbruised fruit; mash well, sieve or liquidise fruit; mix to smooth purée.
Vegetables	
✓	Potato, carrot, swede, turnip, parsnip, cauliflower, tinned vegetables in water only, e.g. carrot, peas.
✖	Fibrous vegetables, e.g. celery, 'long' beans which are difficult to purée.
P	Prepare in usual way and cook in unsalted water, then purée.
Pulses	
✓	Can be used between four and six months, although not generally offered as 'first' food. Lentils, split peas most suitable for smooth purée. Good source of iron.
✖	Pulses with tough skins.
P	Cook well in unsalted water then purée.

Continued

✓ = suitable   ✖ = unsuitable   **P** = preparation

Meat/chicken	
✓	Cooked lamb, beef, chicken. Not generally used as a very 'first food', but can be given as acceptance of new tastes develops. Excellent source of iron. Introduction at this stage is of benefit.
✖	Undercooked meat or meat unsuitable for purée; meat products.
P	Purée well-cooked, plain meat.
Milk products	
✓	Unsweetened natural yoghurt (whole milk if available), unsweetened fromage frais, if thinned. Moving on to: cheese sauce (no added salt), home-made unsweetened custard. 'Baby' yoghurt desserts may be used, but some can be very sweet.
✖	Sweetened yoghurts, unpasteurised milk products, packet sauce mixes, tinned custard, cow's milk as a drink.
Cereals, starchy foods	
✓	First cereals should be gluten-free, e.g. baby rice, cooked ground rice, maize or millet cereals.
✖	Mothers choosing to avoid gluten: wheat, oats, barley, rye cereals, most rusks, some dried infant meals.
P	Mix with infant milk and/or cooled, boiled water.

6.6 The second stage: 6–9 months

6.6.1 Quantity

The quantity of food accepted varies greatly between babies so parents can only be advised accordingly. However, babies should not be force-fed and large quantities of low energy weaning foods (e.g. fruit, vegetables) should be particularly discouraged. Encourage gradual progression towards a pattern of three meals per day.

6.6.2 Consistency

By six months, infants should be offered textured food and soft lumps. Failure to do so may lead to refusal to eat 'lumps' and a disinclination to chew.

Consistency should move gradually from soft lumps to a mashed texture. Finger foods given from around seven months encourage chewing. Suitable finger foods include toast fingers, cheese cubes, vegetable sticks. Rusks are not recommended owing to the sugar content of most varieties.

6.6.3   Salt and sugar

Salt should not be added to food or cooking water, but from 7–8 months a small amount of salt in cooked dishes is not a cause for concern. Very salty foods such as stock cubes, meat or yeast extract and dried sauce mixes are not recommended.

Sugar should not be added to foods except to make sour fruits palatable, and attention should be drawn to the fact that honey, fructose, syrup, malt extract and concentrated fruit juices are as harmful as sugar to incoming teeth.

Artificial sweeteners
Artificial sweeteners should not be added to an infant's food (see Section 24.3.1). These are not permitted in manufactured baby foods.

6.6.4   Foods to include

From six months onwards most foods, including those of higher potential allergenicity, can be given if texture is suitably modified, as shown in Table 6.2. Unpasteurised milk products and other 'high risk' foods should be avoided throughout the first two years (see Chapter 11 – Food Safety).

Table 6.2 Suitable foods and their texture.

Eggs	Hard cooked only
Fish	Bone free
Nuts	As ground nuts or smooth nut butters only
Citrus fruits	With pips removed
Wheat	In bread, crackers, Weetabix etc.
Whole cow's milk	On cereal or in dishes but *not* as a drinking milk

6.6.5   Variety

From six months onwards, solid food makes a significant contribution to nutrient intake. Encouraging as varied a diet as possible is the best means of ensuring an adequate intake of all nutrients. Because different foods supply different combinations of nutrients and certain types of food are good sources of specific nutrients, foods can be classified into groups according to the nutrients they provide, as shown in Fig. 6.1.

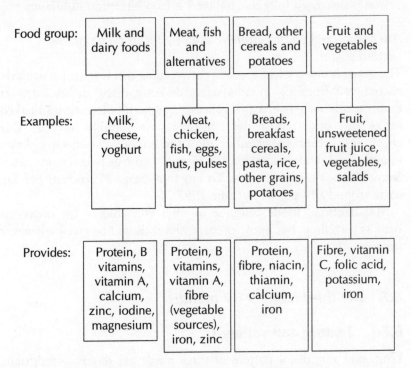

Fig. 6.1 From six months onwards foods should be eaten from each of these groups every day. *From: The National Food Guide. The Balance of Good Health* (HEA 1994).

Fatty and sugary foods?

Some fatty foods such as butter, margarine and oils can be useful sources of vitamins A, D and E and essential fatty acids. Many fatty and sugary foods are of low nutritional value and are therefore considered to be dietary 'extras'. Examples of 'extras' are sweets, cakes, crisps, chocolate and sweet drinks. Dietary variety is an important concept and considered further in Chapter 13 – Assessing Dietary Adequacy.

6.6.6 Iron

An inadequate intake of iron-rich foods during weaning is thought to be one reason for the high rates of iron deficiency found in young children in Britain. Many commercial weaning foods are fortified with iron, but parents need information about foods naturally rich in iron to enable long-term dietary adequacy.

Iron is discussed fully in Chapter 7 – Iron Nutrition in Infancy.

Are home-cooked or commercial baby foods better at this second stage?

The use of home-cooked foods in the weaning diet is to be particularly encouraged from six months onwards since many dishes eaten at family meals such as macaroni cheese, spaghetti bolognese and baked beans can be given if the consistency is suitably altered. This encourages acceptance of 'adult' food and is more cost-effective. As an infant's food intake increases, the financial cost of reliance on manufactured foods is considerable. To buy four 'Stage 2' products per day costs around £18 per week (June 1997).

Manufactured foods continue to offer convenience for occasions such as travelling, but home-prepared food should be given whenever suitable.

6.7   The third stage: 9–12 months

6.7.1   Texture and variety

From nine months, a pattern of three meals per day is appropriate. Food should progress from mashed to minced to finely chopped texture. 'Finger foods' should be given, and by this stage a wide variety of foods should be eaten unless there is a required dietary restriction.

6.7.2   'Family foods'

Giving infants home-prepared foods is to be encouraged, but the terms 'family foods' and 'family meals' can be misleading and need careful use. Changing national eating patterns mean that foods eaten regularly in many households are unsuitable for weaning infants. Foods commonly described as 'convenience foods' are often high in salt or sugar, low in vitamins, and/or very high in fat. Convenience foods which are unsuitable for infants include pastry savouries, pot noodles, deep fried food, sugary cereals and 'take-away' meals (Chinese, Indian etc.).

However, some 'convenience' foods are useful, economical and nutritious. Convenience foods which are suitable for infants include baked beans, spaghetti hoops, tinned vegetables and tinned fruit in unsweetened juice. Convenience ready-made meals are considered in Chapter 23 – Meals and Snacks. Parents' understanding of the term 'family foods' and the use of convenience foods need to be assessed individually. Use of any appropriate family foods should be encouraged.

6.8   Drinks during weaning

As the intake of solid food increases, drinks of cooled, boiled water should be given according to thirst. There is no need to give baby juices but if a mother insists on doing so, these should be as dilute as possible so that the water is barely coloured. Drinking time must always be kept short (see Chapter 10 – Dental Health) and even giving diluted fruit juice from a bottle is not recommended.

6.9   Vegetarian weaning

See Chapter 18 for discussion of vegetarian and ethnic minority diets.

6.9.1   Definitions

The meaning of the term 'vegetarian' must be clarified on an individual basis with parents, as shown in Table 6.3. The term is used here to mean lacto-ovo vegetarian.

Table 6.3   Definitions of 'vegetarian'.

Lacto-ovo vegetarian	Excludes all meat, fish, poultry. Milk products and eggs are still consumed.
Lacto vegetarian	Excludes all meat, fish, poultry and eggs. Milk and milk products are still consumed.
Vegan	Consumes no foods of animal origin.

6.9.2   Vegetarian weaning diet

A vegetarian weaning diet is little different from any other in the first weeks and suitable 'first foods' are the same, i.e. puréed fruit and vegetables, baby rice, gluten-free cereals. As weaning progresses, nutrients at potential risk of insufficiency include energy, iron, good quality protein and vitamin D. General advice can be given as follows.

Energy

- Maintain breast milk, or infant milk feeding, throughout the first year
- Include energy-dense foods, e.g. nut butter, ground nuts and cheese, regularly
- Use less bulky, low fibre cereals as well as high fibre varieties and do not give excessive quantities of fruit and vegetables
- Regular weighing provides a means of monitoring energy intake

Iron

- Give iron-rich foods daily (see Chapter 7) and give vitamin C rich fruit, vegetables or well diluted fruit juice with meals to maximise iron absorption
- Avoid giving tea or excessive quantities of wholegrain cereals which may inhibit iron absorption

Protein

- Include a variety of cereals, pulses and dairy products to achieve a good protein intake (see Chapter 18 – Vegetarian and Ethnic Minority Diets)

Vitamins

- Vegetarian mothers who are breastfeeding should receive vitamin D supplements, and government vitamin supplements are advisable for all vegetarian infants
- Advice should be sought from a dietitian if there is any doubt about the adequacy of a infant's vegetarian diet

6.9.3   Vegan weaning

A vegan diet is highly restrictive and carries considerable risk of nutritional deficiency, including energy, protein, calcium, iron, Vitamins B_{12} and D.

What general advice can I give?
General advice is not sufficient for this group.

Parents choosing to wean their infants on to a vegan diet should receive advice from a dietitian. Additional vitamin supplements may be required.

Interim advice may be given concerning:

- Recommendation of government vitamin drops for all vegan infants and vitamin D for breastfeeding mothers
- Caution regarding dietary bulk
- Continued breastfeeding or use of chosen soya formula throughout the first year
- Regular intake of iron-rich foods and vitamin C-rich foods (see Chapter 7).
- Vitamin B_{12} supplements for breastfeeding mothers.

Note that unmodified soya 'milk' in cartons, and goat's or ewe's milk, must not be given to vegan infants (see Chapter 8).

6.10 What constitutes a nutritionally adequate weaning diet?

Weaning is recognised to be a time of nutritional risk. Nutritional adequacy is most likely to be achieved if foods are chosen each day from each of the four food groups shown in Table 6.4 each day. Adult

Table 6.4 A guide to daily servings from the food groups.

	Milk and dairy foods	Meat, fish and alternatives	Bread, other cereals and potatoes	Fruit and vegetables
6–9 months	500–600 ml breast milk or infant milk Other milk/ milk products in meals	1(+) daily	2–3 daily	2 daily
9–12 months	500–600 ml breast milk or infant milk + other milk/milk products	Minimum 1–2 daily	3–4 daily	3–4 daily

From: Weaning and the Weaning Diet (DoH, 1994).

healthy eating guidelines cannot be applied to young children; this is considered in more detail in Chapter 13. Since it is very difficult to determine accurately nutritional adequacy, infants causing concern must be referred to a dietitian for full dietary assessment. Table 6.4 is a guide to daily 'servings' from each food group.

6.10.1 Checklist for an adequate weaning diet

(1) Foods from each of the food groups daily
(2) 600 ml breast milk or infant milk daily
(3) Vitamin drops if exclusively breastfed after six months, or any dietary restriction
(4) Iron-rich foods daily
(5) Vitamin C rich foods at mealtimes
(6) Limited use of high fibre foods
(7) Restricted use of 'low-fat' foods
(8) Three meals and two snacks from around nine months

Dietary adequacy is considered in detail in Chapter 13.

7. Iron Nutrition in Infancy

> 'It is a matter of concern that diets commonly used during weaning may provide inadequate absorbable iron.'
>
> Weaning and the Weaning Diet, DoH, 1994

This chapter covers:

- The difference between haem iron and non-haem iron
- Sources of iron in a weaning diet
- Foods which promote and inhibit iron absorption
- Advice on achieving an adequate intake of iron during weaning

7.1 Importance of iron in the weaning diet

Term infants are born with sufficient iron stores to last 4–6 months. Iron requirements increase from four months and from this age iron-containing foods need to be supplied in the weaning diet. Breast milk contains little iron, but absorption is excellent. Infant milk has a very high iron content which compensates for poor absorption.

A poor iron intake risks iron deficiency in later infancy and toddler years (1–3 years) and since iron deficiency is often sub-clinical, it may be difficult to detect. Iron status is assessed with reference to definitions set by the World Health Organisation (WHO, 1972).

Anaemia: haemoglobin < 110 g/litre
Iron deficiency: serum ferritin < 10 µg/litre

7.1.1 Why is iron deficiency a cause for concern?

Iron is essential to the oxygen carrying role of haemoglobin and to the metabolism of many organs, including the brain. Iron deficiency anaemia in toddlers is known to be associated with developmental delay, poor growth and weight gain and with recurrent infections.

7.2 Prevalence of iron deficiency

A number of studies have found a high prevalence of anaemia in British toddlers and older infants (Erhardt, 1986; Marder *et al.*, 1990).

Children from Asian communities and areas of social deprivation are known to be at particularly high risk. The National Diet and Nutrition Survey of children aged $1\frac{1}{2}$ to $4\frac{1}{2}$ years (Gregory *et al.*, 1995) found that in a nationally representative sample of almost 1,700 children:

- 12% of children aged $1\frac{1}{2}$–$2\frac{1}{2}$ years were anaemic
- 28% of children aged $1\frac{1}{2}$–$2\frac{1}{2}$ years had serum ferritin below 10 µg/l

Why may iron status be poor?

The major causes of iron deficiency during infancy are dietary (DoH, 1994). Dietary inadequacy may persist into early childhood.

Dietary causes include:

- Early use of cow's milk (before 12 months) as a drinking milk
- Early weaning
- Prolonged milk drinking
- Delayed weaning
- Giving solids close to breast feeds
- Weaning diet contains insufficient iron-rich foods
- Poor intake of vitamin C rich foods
- Lack of awareness of factors affecting iron absorption

Parents need advice about dietary sources of iron and factors affecting iron absorption from the start of weaning to ensure long-term adequacy.

How much iron is required?

Iron requirements in early childhood are high relative to food intake and body size (Table 7.1). For infants, it is equivalent to the amount of iron found in a 250 g portion of minced beef, i.e. a lot of iron!

Table 7.1 Reference Nutrient Intake (RNI).

Infants:	0–3 months	= 7.8 mg/day
	4–6 months	= 4.3 mg/day
	7–12 months	= 7.8 mg/day
Children:	1–3 years	= 6.9 mg/day

7.3   Iron absorption

An individual's iron absorption varies according to iron status. Poor iron status results in greater iron absorption. The efficiency with which iron is absorbed from food and used by the body is described as iron **bioavailability**. Iron bioavailability is determined by the source of iron and its interaction with other foods in the diet.

7.3.1   Types of iron

Foods contain iron in one of two forms: haem iron and non-haem iron. **Haem iron** is found in meat, poultry and fish. **Non-haem iron** is found in some plant foods, e.g. green vegetables, cereals and nuts.

The bioavailability of haem iron is good and is not affected by dietary factors, but the bioavailability of non-haem iron is much more variable because of the way it is bound in foods. Bioavailability of non-haem iron is influenced by dietary factors.

7.3.2   Factors promoting absorption of non-haem iron

The following promote absorption of non-haem iron:

- *Vitamin C*: high in citrus fruit, citrus fruit juices, kiwi fruit, black currants, some vegetables, e.g. peas.
- *Animal protein*: meat, poultry (chicken).

These foods should be consumed at the same time as non-haem iron.

Example
The meal in Table 7.2 allows maximum absorption of iron.

Table 7.2 Example of meal allowing maximum absorption of iron.

Food	Supplies
Minced beef	haem iron
Peas	non-haem iron, vitamin C
Potato	(some) vitamin C
Satsuma	vitamin C

7.3.3   Factors inhibiting absorption of non-haem iron

Table 7.3 shows substances that inhibit absorption of non-haem iron.

The absorption of iron from breast milk is reduced if solids are given close to a feed. Inhibitors in the food bind the iron, making it less available. Intake of nutritious foods containing inhibitors (e.g. pulses, eggs) should not be discouraged if given at a different time from a breast feed. These foods themselves provide useful amounts of iron.

Table 7.3   Substances inhibiting absorption of non-haem iron.

Substance	Found in
Tannin	Tea, legumes
Non-starch polysaccharide (NSP) (fibre)	Wholemeal products
Phytic acid	Unrefined cereals, e.g. brown rice, bran, pulses
Phosphates	Eggs, some plant foods
Oxalates	Rhubarb, spinach
Polyphenols	Spinach, coffee

7.4   Sources of iron in the weaning diet

Iron is obtained from:

- Breast milk or infant milk
- Iron-rich foods, e.g. red meat, green leafy vegetables
- Iron fortified infant foods, e.g. baby rice, 'Stage I' meals, rusks
- Other iron fortified foods, e.g. breakfast cereals

Cow's milk and milk products are low in iron. Whole cow's milk is therefore not recommended as a main (drinking) milk before one year (DoH, 1994) (see Chapter 8). Follow-on milk is fortified with iron and may be used. However, it is not routinely recommended since breast milk and infant milk are suitable up to one year.

The contribution of a food to iron intake depends not only on iron bioavailability (see above), but also on the frequency with which it is eaten. It can be misleading to think of a food as a 'very good' source of iron if it is eaten infrequently.

The survey *The Food and Nutrient Intakes of British Infants Aged 6–12 months* (Mills & Tyler, 1992) considered the contribution of different foods to daily iron intakes at age 9–12 months (Table 7.4). This illustrates the role of fortified infant foods as a nutritional 'safety net' for infants. Over-reliance on such foods is to be avoided, however, since it is only increased awareness and use of 'adult' foods that ensure a good iron intake beyond infancy and early childhood.

Table 7.4 Contribution of different foods to daily iron intakes at age 9–12 months.

Food	% contribution to iron intake
Meats	7%
Breakfast cereals	13%
'Other foods'	30%
Fortified infant foods, infant milk	50%

A comprehensive list of iron-containing foods is given in Section 13.4.2. Table 7.5 is a suggested guide to the introduction of iron-containing foods during weaning.

Foods which are 'not recommended', but may contribute a significant amount of iron are: rusks, chocolate and chocolate products, biscuits.

7.4.1 Iron for vegetarian infants

A good intake of foods containing non-haem iron and vitamin C, to promote iron absorption, is important for vegetarian infants. Many of the foods listed previously are suitable in a vegetarian diet. Some of those in Table 7.6 should be eaten regularly. Consistency of foods should, of course, be modified according to age.

High fibre vegetarian diets inhibit iron absorption. Referral should be made to a dietitian if there is any doubt about dietary adequacy.

Table 7.5 Suggested timetable for use of foods containing iron.

	4–6 months	6–8 months	9 months +
Meat, fish and alternatives	Plain meat, e.g. chicken, turkey; pulses, e.g. lentils. 'Stage 1' infant meals.	Boned white fish, hard cooked eggs, quorn. Baked beans, smooth peanut butter, ground nuts, 'Stage 2' infant meals.	Bone-free tinned fish, e.g. tuna. Limited use of higher salt foods, e.g. corned beef, meat or fish paste.
Bread, other cereals	Baby rice, gluten-free infant cereals.	Weetabix-type cereal. Bread, plain crackers, (rusk – see text).	Breakfast cereals, e.g. Rice Krispies.
Vegetables and fruit	Puréed green non-fibrous vegetables: spring greens, broccoli, peas, watercress etc. Dried fruit purée.	Greater variety of green vegetables.	Any
Milk* and dairy foods	Breast milk. Infant milks. Infant formulae.	Follow-on milk if necessary.	

*Cow's milk is *not* rich in iron.

7.5 Practical questions

What can I advise to ensure an adequate iron intake?

- Give breast milk or infant milk as the 'main' drinking milk until one year
- Start weaning at 4–6 months
- Give foods containing haem iron daily (if acceptable)
- Include green vegetables in the diet from an early age
- Give vitamin C rich fruit, or well diluted fruit juice at mealtimes

Table 7.6 Foods to be eaten regularly by vegetarian infants.

Food	Example	From (months)
Pulses	Lentils, chick peas, butter beans, mung beans.	4+
Soya products	Tofu, textured vegetable protein (TVP) Burger type products.	6+ 9+
Nuts	Ground, or in butters: smooth peanut butter, almond, cashew.	6+
Seeds	Ground sesame, pumpkin, sunflower.	6+
Eggs	Hard cooked.	6+
Quorn	Plain variety.	6+
Cereals	Infant rice cereals, millet. Wheat, oats, other gluten-containing cereals.	4+ 6+
Dried fruit	Apricots, prunes, figs.	4+

- Use fortified (infant and then adult) cereals
- Avoid tea or a diet high in fibre

Should iron supplements be given?

Iron supplements are used where there is proven iron deficiency but are not generally recommended as a prophylactic measure. Compliance in giving iron drops is poor and there is recent evidence to suggest that in the absence of deficiency an excessive iron intake can retard growth (Idjradinata *et al.*, 1993).

What about screening for iron deficiency?

Screening programmes for iron deficiency in toddlers have been set up in a few areas, e.g. Bradford and Bristol. Iron status is determined from a finger prick blood sample. Programmes of this kind are not widespread and there is considerable debate as to the cost implications, viability and desirability of a national screening strategy. The health professional is well placed, however, to identify infants and young children at risk of iron deficiency given that most contributory factors are dietary (see Section 7.2). Pre-term and Asian infants are also at increased risk of iron deficiency and families should be given dietary advice routinely.

Assessment of iron intake is discussed in Section 13.4.2.

8.   Cow's Milk and Other Milks

'Pasteurised whole cow's milk should only be used as a main milk drink after the age of one year.'

Weaning and the Weaning Diet, DoH, 1994

This chapter covers:

- Advice on the introduction and appropriate use of whole cow's milk in an infant's diet
- The differences between follow-on milks and standard infant milks
- The specialist nature of soya infant formula

Milk is a dietary staple of major nutritional significance throughout infancy, but mothers need advice concerning the role of different milks.

8.1   Cow's milk

8.1.1   Use of cow's milk

Cow's milk has a very different composition to human breast milk and is not suitable for a young infant.

'Pasteurised whole cow's milk should only be used as a main milk drink after the age of one year'.

Weaning and the Weaning Diet (DoH, 1994)

The appropriate use of cow's milk requires consideration of:

- Potential renal solute load
- Allergenicity
- Iron content
- Vitamin D content
- Potential gastrointestinal blood loss

Renal solute load
Cow's milk has a higher protein and sodium content than breast milk

and therefore a higher renal solute load. Kidney function and the ability to concentrate urine is immature in a young infant. A renal solute load in excess of capacity may increase water lost in the urine with the potential for dehydration.

Allergenicity

Cow's milk protein is recognised to be allergenic. Risk of allergy is increased in young infants because the gut is more permeable to food allergens, and infants of atopic parents are at greatest risk (see Chapter 9 – Food Intolerance and Allergy).

Introduction of cow's milk and cow's milk products before six months should be strongly discouraged for infants of atopic parents.

Iron content

Cow's milk contains little iron, which is of low availability. Iron requirements are increased in late infancy, and must be supplied by dietary intake once birth stores are depleted (see Section 7.1 – Importance of iron). Early use of cow's milk as a main source of milk has been identified as a risk factor for iron deficiency (Mills, 1990).

Vitamin D

Cow's milk contains little vitamin D. Skin synthesis of vitamin D shows seasonal variability and infants fed cow's milk as a main drinking milk may be at risk of vitamin D deficiency, unless government vitamin drops are given. Asian and Afro-Caribbean infants having cow's milk as a drinking milk are at particularly high risk of vitamin D deficiency.

Gastrointestinal blood loss

A small amount of gastrointestinal blood loss in infants is recognised as quite normal (Anyon & Clarkson, 1969). A few studies have found that the use of cow's milk in infant diets can cause increased blood loss, but the methodology of these studies has been called into question.

When can cow's milk be given to an infant?

Gut maturity is achieved 3–4 months post term. In **non-allergic** infants the introduction of cow's milk should be based on digestive and nutritional considerations and not on those of potential allergenicity (American Academy of Pediatrics, 1992).

Delayed introduction of cow's milk and other common food allergens

beyond six months is advisable for infants from strongly atopic families (Cant & Bailes, 1984; DoH, 1994).

Current recommendations propose that whole cow's milk can be given to non-allergenic infants, as shown in Table 8.1.

Table 8.1   Whole cow's milk given to non-allergenic infants.

Aged from	Given as
4 months*	Milk-containing solids, e.g. cheese, unsweetened yoghurts, custard
6 months	To mix cereals
12 months	As a main drinking milk

Pasteurised whole cow's milk should only be used as a main drink after the age of one year (DoH, 1994).

This recommendation is based on concern about the low iron and vitamin D content of cow's milk and reflects current expert opinion. The distinction made between the use of cow's milk **'products'** at four months and the use of whole cow's milk at six months is a potential source of confusion. It is based on the **amount** of cow's milk involved.

The 1990 OPCS survey of infant feeding (White *et al.*, 1992) found that:

- 11% of mothers gave whole cow's milk as the main milk before six months
- 36% of mothers gave whole cow's milk as the main milk before nine months

These figures show significant improvement from the previous survey in 1985.

Why do mothers give whole cow's milk as the main milk at such a young age?
The decision is influenced by:

- Cost considerations
- Parental and peer group influence
- Convenience
- Inconsistent professional advice

Confusion amongst professionals as to the appropriate use of cow's milk in infancy is a recognised problem (Hyde, 1994).

What can I advise for an infant given cow's milk as a drink earlier than recommended?

- Use of breast milk, infant milk or, after six months of age, follow-on milk as a drinking milk, with continued additional use of whole cow's milk/products

If this is unacceptable:

- Use of whole milk only, and not reduced fat varieties (see next section).
- Use of undiluted milk. Diluting will compromise energy intake. Renal solute load is increased by feeding cow's milk, but in the majority of older infants, renal capacity is unlikely to be exceeded.
- Supplementary vitamin drops, given daily in the recommended dose of five drops.
- Daily inclusion of iron-fortified and iron-rich foods in the diet (see Chapter 7 – Iron Nutrition).

8.1.2   Reduced fat milk

The OPCS survey of 1990 found that of parents who gave their infants cow's milk:

- 7% gave reduced fat milk as the main drinking milk
- 21% gave reduced fat milk as a second milk, in cooking

Reduced fat milk (semi-skimmed or skimmed) should *not* be given to an infant, even if it is used by the rest of the family.

Why are reduced fat milks unsuitable for infants?
Whole milk is an important source of energy and other nutrients in a young child's diet. Childhood energy requirements per unit of body weight are highest during the first year of life and, because stomach capacity is small, an infant's diet must supply a lot of energy in a small volume of food. The energy density of whole milk is therefore appropriate for infant and toddler needs. Whole milk additionally supplies fat soluble vitamins A, D and E, not found in significant amounts in reduced fat milks.

The adoption of healthy eating habits is to be encouraged in a young child, but inappropriate restriction of dietary fat may lead to poor growth and is not appropriate in the first two years of life.

Semi-skimmed milk may be introduced from two years of age, if energy and nutrient intake is otherwise adequate and growth remains satisfactory (DoH, 1994).

However, skimmed milk should not be given to a child under five years of age.

8.2   Follow-on milk

Follow-on milk has a higher iron and vitamin D content than other infant milks. However, it should only be given to an infant from six months and is unsuitable for younger infants because compared to breast milk and other infant milks:

- It is compositionally closer to cow's milk
- It generally has a higher protein and sodium content which increases the renal solute load

Follow-on milks are not available under the welfare system for families on low incomes.

Table 8.2 shows available brands of follow-on milks. Follow-on milks are not intended to replace breast milk or infant milks which are recommended until at least 12 months. However, follow-on milks are nutritionally more suitable than cow's milk and are therefore useful for those mothers who wish to move on and would otherwise use cow's milk.

Follow-on milks are fortified with iron, and a child's iron status may be compromised once this milk is no longer used. Therefore mothers must be made aware of the need for iron and how to include iron-rich foods in the weaning diet (Wharton, 1990; DoH, 1994).

Table 8.2   Brands of follow-on milks (June 1997).

Cow and Gate Step Up
Farleys Follow-on Milk
Milupa Forward
SMA Progress
Sainsbury's First Menu: Follow-on Milk
Boots Junior Milk

Follow-on milk is not suitable for infants under six months of age (DoH, 1994).

8.3   Goat's milk

Goat's milk should not be given to infants (DoH, 1994) because:

- Goat's milk is not nutritionally complete; levels of vitamins A, D and C and folic acid are low. Feeding with goat's milk has been associated with infant megaloblastic anaemia.
- Goat's milk is not subject to the same hygiene legislation as cow's milk, and can be bought unpasteurised. Unpasteurised goat's milk is a potential source of salmonella and brucellosis infection.
- Goat's milk has a potentially high renal solute load.
- There is no evidence to suggest that goat's milk reduces the risk of allergic disease. This is unlikely because cow and goat milk protein are very similar.

If parents insist on feeding goat's milk:

- Recommend use of a pasteurised product only, or at least boiling the milk for two minutes to reduce risk of microbiological contamination.
- Ensure a folic acid supplement is given, under medical supervision (average folic acid requirement is 40 µg per day in infancy).
- Ensure government vitamin supplements in the recommended dose of five drops per day are given from one month of age.
- Monitor growth closely.
- If there is any doubt about nutritional adequacy, refer to a dietitian for dietary assessment.

8.4   Ewe's milk

Like goat's milk, ewe's milk is not suitable for infants (DoH, 1994). The use of ewe's milk should be discouraged for the same reasons as goat's milk: it is nutritionally incomplete, it has a high renal solute load, and it may be microbiologically unsafe.

Also like goat's milk, ewe's milk is not thought to be any less allergenic than cow's milk.

Folic acid supplements must be given to any infant fed ewe's or goat's milk. Government supplementary vitamin drops are required from one month of age.

8.5 Soya infant formula

Soya infant formula is manufactured from soya protein isolate and is nutritionally complete. It is free from cow's milk and therefore suitable for some infants requiring a cow's milk free diet (see Section 9.8). Table 8.3 shows available brands of soya infant formula.

Table 8.3 Brands of soya infant formula (June 1997).

Abbott Laboratories Isomil
Cow and Gate Infasoy
Heinz Soya Formula
Mead Johnson Prosobee
SMA Wysoy

Soya infant formula is not an appropriate substitute for breast milk unless there is a specific need to exclude cow's milk from the diet. Feeding soya infant formula has not been found to protect against the development of allergic disease (Miskelly *et al.*, 1988). Casual use of soya infant formula in response to vague symptoms may delay diagnosis of underlying disease.

8.5.1 Dental health

Lactose is the naturally occurring sugar in human and cow's milk and is also the predominant sugar in most infant formulae. Soya infant formulae contain glucose syrups as an alternative sugar and are therefore lactose free and suitable for infants who are lactose intolerant. Glucose syrups are manufactured from the hydrolysis of corn starch and are a mixture of glucose, maltose and longer chain saccharides.

There is concern that soya infant formulae are potentially more cariogenic than standard infant formulae because they contain glucose syrups, but the acidogenicity of soya infant formulae has not been found to be statistically different from infant milks (Moynihan *et al.*, 1996). However, the frequency and duration of feeds of soya infant formula and whether the feeds are from a bottle or at bed time is likely to have a marked effect on cariogenicity. Consequently, for dental health purposes, infants should be encouraged to drink from a cup by six months, they should not be left with milk-containing bottles as comforters and milk feeds at bedtime should be discouraged.

8.5.2 Aluminium

Aluminium is ubiquitous in nature and found in variable amounts in soil, water and foods. It is non-toxic, except where renal function is impaired when bone accumulation may occur. Higher levels of aluminium have been found in soya infant formula than in standard infant milk although the levels are still low relative to the current guidelines of 7 mg/kg/week established by WHO. However, these formulae are not recommended for premature infants or those suffering from renal failure.

8.5.3 Phytoestrogens

There has been concern expressed about the presence of phytoestrogens in soya infant formulae because they can behave like a weak form of the female hormone oestrogen. Phytoestrogens occur naturally in the soya protein used in soya infant formulae. Some types of phytoestrogens, i.e. coumestans, which are not found in soya, have been shown to cause infertility in animals. Work is underway which will give a better understanding of how the phytoestrogens in soya behave in humans since these actions are complex and are not understood.

Infants who are cow's milk intolerant or vegans may continue to be given soya infant formulae (SODH/CMO, 1996).

8.6 Soya 'milk'

Soya 'milk' in cartons, available from supermarkets and health food shops, must not be given to infants. These products do not contain sufficient energy, minerals or vitamins to support infant growth.

8.7 Role of milk in the weaning diet

All recommended milks (i.e. breast milk, infant milk, whole cow's milk, follow-on milk) provide energy, protein, calcium and B vitamins in a weaning diet. Breast milk, infant milk and follow-on milk provide iron and vitamin D, but whole cow's milk is a poor source of these nutrients.

How much milk should be given?

Throughout the first year a minimum of 500–600 ml (1 pint approx.) of breast milk or infant milk should be given daily as the main drinking milk. In addition to this, whole cow's milk may be used on cereals from six months onwards.

Can an infant consume too much milk?

Milk is a valuable source of nutrients but excessive consumption may limit appetite for other foods, and long-term dietary adequacy is dependent on consumption of a wide variety of foods. In the second half of infancy total milk intake should therefore be limited to about 800 ml ($1\frac{1}{2}$ pints) per day.

What if an infant refuses all forms of milk?

Food refusal is common in young children and is discussed fully in Chapters 16 and 21 – Feeding Problems)

An intake of 500–600 ml of breast milk or infant milk per day in the first year ensures that calcium requirements for bone mineralisation are met. Where milk 'as a drink' is refused, suggest giving:

- More milk in cooking, e.g. porridge, cheese sauce, custard, rice pudding
- Milk products, e.g. yoghurt (avoid low fat varieties), cheese, fromage frais
- Flavoured milk drinks, e.g. milk blended with banana, tinned fruit in natural juice or fruit yoghurt

Sweetened milk drinks should never be given from a bottle. Adequate care must be taken in respect of dental health if sweetened milk drinks are given.

For further food sources of calcium see Section 13.4.1.

An infant who persists in refusing milk and milk products may require calcium supplements, and should be referred to a dietitian for dietary assessment.

9. Food Intolerance and Allergy

> 'Food allergy as a topic has been plagued by misunderstanding and confusion for years.'
>
> Bock *et al.*, 1979

This chapter covers:

- The difference between food allergy and intolerance
- The need for specialist advice in cases of suspected food intolerance
- Factors increasing an infant's risk of food intolerance

9.1 Definitions

The term 'allergy' is widely misused. Adverse reactions to food are common, but only a minority are due to allergic reactions. The following definitions were adopted in a 1984 joint report of the Royal College of Physicians and British Nutrition Foundation (RCP/BNF, 1984):

- *Food intolerance* – Reproducible, unpleasant reaction to food which is not psychologically based. Occurs even when food is given in disguised form.
- *Food allergy* – Form of food intolerance in which there is clear evidence of an abnormal immunological reaction to the food.
- *Food aversion* – Avoidance of food due to psychological reasons.

Other terms requiring clarification include (David, 1993):

- *Antigen* – Substance capable of provoking an immune response. Usually a protein, but may be a polysaccharide (carbohydrate).
- *Antibody* – Immunoglobulin (protein) able to combine specifically with certain antigens.
- *Allergen* – Substance which provokes a harmful immune response, i.e. allergic response.

9.2 Reactions to food

9.2.1 Food allergy

Food allergy always involves an immunological response. Food allergy involves **sensitisation** to food and a number of factors contribute to risk of sensitisation. The process of sensitisation in the susceptible infant is:

Food antigen ingested → crosses gut wall → specific antibody produced = sensitisation

Further contact with the same food antigen triggers an active adverse response by the immune system, i.e. an allergic reaction.

9.2.2 Non-allergenic food intolerance

Food intolerant reactions not involving an immunological response may result from:

- Enzyme deficiency, e.g. lactose intolerance
- Pharmacological effect, e.g. caffeine, vasoactive amines
- Irritant effect on mucous membranes, e.g. very spicy curries
- Fermentation of unabsorbed food in lower bowel

9.3 Foods causing intolerant reactions

Virtually any food can cause symptoms of intolerance but foods most commonly associated with intolerance in children are:

- Cow's milk
- Eggs
- Wheat
- Nuts (especially peanuts)
- Soya
- Citrus fruit

9.4 Prevalence

Accurate information concerning the prevalence of food intolerance and allergy in children is lacking but between 0.3 and 20% of children are thought to have been affected by some form of intolerance (RCP/BNF, 1984). It is also known that:

- Allergy runs in families: a child of atopic parents is at increased risk (see Section 9.7).
- The prevalence of food allergy and intolerance is greatest in the first few months of life.

Intolerance to milk and eggs in particular resolves with increasing age.

Why is this estimate so approximate?

The range of reported figures reflects the many factors which confound the study of allergic disease in children. These include the difficulties in distinguishing between food intolerance and systemic disease, a lack of definite diagnostic tests, differing diagnostic criteria of various studies, the subjective nature of symptom recall and diagnosis by parents.

9.5   Symptoms

Food intolerance and allergy in infants and children are associated with a wide range of symptoms, as shown in Table 9.1. Symptoms vary widely in their time of onset and severity and several different symptoms may coexist. In spite of a widely held public perception, behavioural symptoms due to food intolerance are uncommon.

Table 9.1 Symptoms of food intolerance and allergy in infants and children.

Symptoms	Examples
Gastrointestinal	Diarrhoea Vomiting Abdominal distension Recurrent bleeding Failure to thrive
Respiratory	Wheezing Rhinitis Asthma Anaphylaxis
Dermatological	Urticaria Eczema
Behavioural	Hyperactivity

9.6 Diagnosis

Diagnosis of food intolerance and allergy is difficult unless there is an acute reaction. Three diagnostic approaches are used: clinical assessment, biochemical testing and dietary elimination.

Clinical assessment

Involves study of symptoms, dietary history and family history of atopic disease.

Biochemical testing

Where an immunologically mediated reaction is suspected, tests can be carried out to detect raised levels of IgE antibodies. Two tests are validated:

- *Radioallergosorbent (RAST) test* – Detects the level of circulating antibodies in response to a food antigen
- *Skin prick test* – Seeks to provoke a skin-based response to a food antigen

Unfortunately, both RAST and skin prick tests lack reliability. False positive results are not uncommon, when antibody levels may be raised but there is no observed adverse reaction to a food. False negative results also occur routinely. The results of IgE tests therefore need to be interpreted with caution, and their diagnostic value is somewhat limited (David, 1993). Unorthodox diagnostic tests such as pulse testing, cytotoxic testing and trace metal hair testing are not recommended. The validity of such tests is unproven.

Dietary elimination and challenge

This requires elimination of an implicated food from the diet to see whether symptoms improve. Any improvement is challenged with reintroduction of the food. Dietary challenge is the best means available of diagnosing food intolerance/allergy (David, 1993) but should be undertaken only under the supervision of a dietitian and paediatrician.

9.7 Risk factors for the development of allergies

Allergies run in families. The risk of a child developing an allergic disorder more than doubles if there is a parent or sibling history of atopic disease (Kjellman, 1977). A raised concentration of IgE anti-bodies detected in an infant's cord blood at birth is also indicative of an infant at risk since this shows an immunological predisposition to allergy.

The infant 'at risk' of allergy has:

- A family history of allergic disease *and/or*
- Raised IgE concentration in the cord blood

Genetic and immunological predisposition are the most important determinants of allergic disease, but these may be modified by:

- Type of milk feeding
- Maternal diet during lactation
- Timing and mode of weaning
- Environmental factors

9.7.1 Type of milk feeding

For infants 'at risk', exclusive breastfeeding for at least 4–6 months may reduce the incidence of allergic disease (Cant, 1991). The reason for this is not known exactly but it may be due to the avoidance of exposure to foreign protein, the down regulation of allergic responses or the protection of gut mucosa integrity. Results of studies in this area have been conflicting and more research is needed.

9.7.2 Maternal diet during lactation

An infant can be sensitised to certain food antigens as a result of their presence in breast milk. If risk is considered to be particularly high, exclusion of common food allergens from the maternal diet may be appropriate (Chandra *et al.*, 1989).

Advice should be sought from a dietitian about maternal dietary exclusion.

9.7.3 Timing and mode of weaning

This area has not been fully investigated and conclusive evidence is lacking. To date evidence suggests that:

- Introduction of solid food before four months of age may be associated with increased risk of eczema, especially in infants with a family history of atopic disease (Fergusson *et al.*, 1990; Forsyth *et al.*, 1993)

- Delayed introduction of common food allergens, e.g. cow's milk, eggs, nuts is beneficial for 'at risk' infants

The interaction between breastfeeding, the delayed introduction of solid food and the incidence of allergic disease is currently being studied.

9.7.4 Environmental factors

Exposure to non-food allergens, e.g. cigarette smoke or contact with pets, is thought to increase susceptible infants' risk of allergy.

What can I advise to prevent food allergy?
This cannot be answered satisfactorily. Risk is strongly influenced by genetic factors (see Section 9.7). For infants 'at risk' the following may be suggested:

- Exclusive breastfeeding for at least four, and possibly six months (Cant & Bailes, 1984)
- Possible maternal dietary exclusion of known allergens (see above)
- Gradual weaning on to less allergenic foods, with foods introduced one at a time
- Delayed introduction of allergenic foods until at least six months. However, there is no justification for recommending soya infant formula as a means of preventing allergy.

Referral should be made to a dietitian if detailed advice is required.

9.8 Cow's milk intolerance

A minority of children suffer adverse symptoms after consumption of cow's milk or milk products. This is most commonly due to intolerance to lactose (milk sugar), and/or to cow's milk protein. Suspected cow's milk intolerance requires specialist management and referral to a paediatrician and dietitian.

9.8.1 Lactose intolerance

Characteristics
Intolerance to lactose results from an insufficiency of the lactose digesting enzyme, lactase. The condition commonly follows gastro-

enteritis, such as that due to rotavirus infection or any condition where gut lining is damaged. Lactose intolerance results in symptoms of diarrhoea with foamy stool, and diagnosis is confirmed by detection of reducing substances in the stool. The condition is transient, lasting from a few weeks to six months, and is treated with a cow's milk free diet.

Incidence

The inability to digest lactose due to lactase insufficiency is racially distributed and is more common among non-white races. Primary lactase insufficiency, however, is uncommon in infancy and early childhood.

Around 7.5% of children with gastroenteritis have been found to develop secondary lactose intolerance (Trounce & Walker-Smith, 1985).

9.8.2   Cow's milk protein intolerance (CMPI)

CMPI is an immunologically based intolerance, i.e. a 'true' allergy. The condition is often associated with gastrointestinal symptoms and gut enteropathy but multiple symptoms are common. CMPI can occasionally cause an acute, anaphylactic reaction.

Reliable diagnosis is made by withdrawal and challenge with cow's milk, and immunological tests are also used. CMPI is treated with a cow's milk free diet and tolerance is usually achieved at between 12 months and 5 years (David, 1993).

Prevalence

Intolerance to cow's milk protein is less common than intolerance to lactose. CMPI is particularly prevalent in infants and pre-school children and is usually transitory. The incidence of CMPI has been estimated to be 2% in the first year (Adler & Warner, 1991).

9.8.3   Dietary management

Any infant with cow's milk intolerance requiring a cow's milk free diet should be referred to a dietitian.

Can breastfeeding continue?

Breastfeeding is suitable for most infants with CMPI but where sensitisation is thought to have occurred via breast milk, maternal dietary exclusion of allergic foods (under dietetic supervision) may be appropriate. Infants with lactose intolerance may not tolerate breast milk because it contains lactose.

Where breastfeeding is not possible, a nutritionally suitable alternative to cow's milk based infant milk must be given and this may be hydrolysed protein infant milk formula (HPF) or soya infant formula.

9.8.4 Hydrolysed protein formula (protein hydrolysate)

These formulae are made from hydrolysed protein (partially broken down) which is derived from casein, whey, soya or beef. The process of hydrolysis greatly reduces protein allergenicity. These formulae are supplemented with vitamins and minerals and are nutritionally complete. Table 9.2 shows available brands of hydrolysed protein formulae.

Table 9.2 Brands of hydrolysed protein formulae (June 1997).

Cow & Gate Pepti-Junior
Mead Johnson Pregestimil
Mead Johnson Nutramigen
Milupa Prejomin
Scientific Hospital Supplies Pepdite 0–2

A hydrolysate formula is the recommended choice of formula for the management of an infant with cow's milk protein intolerance (Carter, 1994). Protein hydrolysate formula is considerably more expensive than soya infant formula and is available on prescription.

9.8.5 Soya infant formula and others

Use of soya infant formula is also considered in Section 8.5.

Soya intolerance may coexist with intolerance to cow's milk protein. It is more common in infants with CMPI; up to 30% of these infants are likely to be sensitised to soya protein (Milla, 1988) and there is no evidence that soya protein is less capable than milk protein of producing gastrointestinal symptoms of intolerance. Soya infant formula is not generally recommended for pre-term infants, or infants with impaired renal function, owing to past concerns about its aluminium content (see Section 8.5.2).

When can soya infant formula be used?

- For most infants with secondary lactose intolerance
- For older infants with non-gastrointestinal symptoms, e.g. eczema
- For infants with primary deficiency of lactose, or galactosaemia
- For vegan infants (see Section 8.5.3)

Parents of infants given soya infant formula require advice about practices to safeguard dental health.

Other infant milk substitutes
The following must *not* be used to replace infant milk:

- Goat's milk
- Ewe's milk
- Soya 'milk' – available in cartons from health food shops and supermarkets

These milks are nutritionally incomplete and unsuitable for infants.

9.8.6   Milk free weaning

Parents should receive advice from a dietitian before starting to wean an infant on to a milk free diet.

Exclusion of all sources of cow's milk, including 'hidden' sources in manufactured foods, is required. A dietitian is able to provide specialist advice and written information on the diet and ensure that it is nutritionally adequate. Delaying the introduction of other common food allergens may also be appropriate.

Does an infant on a milk free diet require vitamin or mineral supplements?
If less than 500 ml of the recommended milk substitute is taken, a calcium and vitamin supplement may be required. If there is any doubt about the nutritional adequacy of an infant's diet, referral should be made to a dietitian.

What can I advise for an infant who refuses to take the milk substitute?
Parental attitude can negatively influence intake; reassurance and encouragement may be helpful. The unpleasant taste is lessened by

chilling and can be masked by use of milk free flavourings. Using the milk substitute to make desserts and sauces may help to boost intake. Recipe booklets are available from a dietitian or some manufacturers of soya infant formulae.

How long will a cow's milk free diet be necessary?

Cow's milk sensitivity usually resolves by the age of five years (David, 1993). The timing and method of reintroduction of cow's milk varies. In cases of lactose intolerance, lactose may be reintroduced by accident or a staged reintroduction carried out after a few months. In cases of cow's milk protein intolerance, challenge is rarely undertaken before 12 months of age and requires medical supervision. A positive reaction can occasionally cause an anaphylactic reaction.

10. Dental Health

> 'Correct nutrition plays the key role in ensuring dental health for children.'
>
> Rugg-Gunn, 1993

This chapter covers:

- The importance of preventive dental health care in infancy
- The process of dental caries
- Dietary sources of non-milk extrinsic sugars
- Simple tooth care advice

10.1 Introduction

Dental disease is a significant health and social problem in Britain yet it is largely preventable. There are two major dental diseases: **periodontal** (gum) **disease** and **dental caries** (tooth decay). Dental caries is the major problem in young children. The risk of dental caries can be greatly reduced by effective parent-targeted dental health education. Establishing good dental habits in infancy and early childhood is central to long-term dental health.

The publications *The Scientific Basis of Dental Health Education* (HEA, 1996) and *A Handbook of Dental Health for Health Visitors* (HEA, 1992) are recommended.

10.2 The prevalence of dental caries

The British Association for the Study of Community Dentistry (BASCD) monitors the prevalence of dental caries in five year old children and highlights the impact of early dental habits on dental health. The prevalence of dental caries in infants is not known, but the condition of 'nursing bottle caries' (decayed primary front teeth) is a recognised problem in many areas.

Prevalence is strongly influenced by social factors. Dental caries is more likely in young children in areas of social deprivation (Cushing & Gelbier, 1988), and in those of Asian origin. Caries experience is also positively correlated with the level of non-milk extrinsic (NME) sugars in the diet (Holt, 1990).

10.3 The process of dental caries

The tooth is made up of three layers:

- *Enamel* – Protective outer shell which is the hardest part
- *Dentine* – Softer, sensitive part beneath the enamel
- *Pulp* – Interior

The process of caries starts when the enamel is attacked and demineralised (softened). The destruction spreads to the dentine and the weakened enamel collapses to form a cavity. This continues eventually to the pulp.

What causes demineralisation?

Dietary sugars are the major cause of demineralisation. Bacteria naturally occurring in the mouth metabolise sugars and produce acid as a by-product of metabolism. When mouth acidity reaches a certain level, calcium and phosphate ions are lost from the tooth enamel, i.e. demineralisation occurs.

Sugars + mouth bacteria (plaque) → acid → demineralisation
= *risk of decay*

10.4 Factors influencing the risk of dental caries

The severity of 'an acid attack' and resulting risk of dental caries is influenced by:

- Saliva
- Plaque
- Frequency and duration of sugar intake
- Type of dietary sugar
- Tooth resistance

10.4.1 Saliva

Saliva acts as a natural buffering agent to neutralise the mouth following acid production. Saliva also supplies calcium and phosphate ions which promote remineralisation of tooth enamel. The process of neutralisation takes 20–40 minutes, but it is inhibited by further consumption of sugars. Saliva production is minimal at night and teeth are therefore vulnerable at this time.

10.4.2   Plaque

Plaque exists as a layer of bacteria on the surface of teeth. The bacteria contribute to acid formation and the plaque layer prevents effective buffering by saliva. Careful brushing can remove about half of the plaque from teeth. Brushing with a mild fluoride toothpaste needs to be started from appearance of the first tooth (see Section 10.5.6).

10.4.3   Frequency of sugar intake

Although the amount of sugar consumed is an important factor in the development of dental decay, the frequency of sugar consumption is of greater significance. Frequent sugar intake promotes repeated acid production by bacteria and prevents the buffering action of saliva.

Frequent NME sugars + mouth bacteria (plaque) → frequent acid → prolonged demineralisation = high risk of decay

Parents must understand the importance of reducing the *frequency* and *duration* of sugar intake by limiting sweetened food and drinks to mealtimes.

10.4.4   Dietary sugars

There are many different dietary sugars. All can be metabolised to acids but some are considered to be more harmful to enamel than others, i.e. more cariogenic. Sugars have been classified on the basis of their availability for metabolism (Fig. 10.1).

Intrinsic sugars are those naturally incorporated into the cellular structure of food, e.g. in whole fruit and vegetables. These are of low cariogencity.

Extrinsic sugars are those found free in food, or added to it, e.g. table sugar, sugars in fruit juice and fruit purée (the cellular structure of the fruit has been broken down), honey. Extrinsic sugars are also found in milk and milk products, i.e. lactose, but milk sugars are of low cariogenicity, and milk itself is almost noncariogenic. Extrinsic sugars other than those in milk are called non-milk extrinsic (NME) sugars.

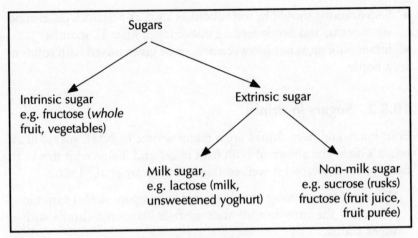

Fig. 10.1 Classification of dietary sugars

Non-milk extrinsic sugars are highly cariogenic. NME sugars include sucrose (table sugar), glucose, fructose.

10.5   Dietary sugars in infancy

The recommended maximum intake of NME sugars for pre-school children is 10% of total dietary energy. NME sugars have been found to provide 9% of dietary energy at 6–9 months and 12% of dietary energy at 9–12 months (Mills & Tyler, 1992).

Where does the sugar in an infant's diet come from?
Sugars are derived from milk, non-milk drinks and many foods. These are considered below.

10.5.1   Sugars in milks

Lactose (milk sugar) is the carbohydrate source in breast milk and most standard infant milks and cow's milk. Lactose is of low cariogenicity. Soya infant formulae, follow-on milks and specialised infant formulae generally contain NME sugars in addition to, or in place of, lactose.

Practical advice about milk feeds

- Although breast milk and infant milk are believed to be of low cariogenicity, feeding times should be finite.
- Comforter bottles should not be given.

- Cup drinking should be introduced as soon as practical, i.e. around six months, and bottle feeding discouraged after 12 months.
- Infant milk must not be sweetened, or be given mixed with solids in a bottle.

10.5.2   Sugars in drinks

Fruit juices and juice drinks are a major source of NME sugars in an infant's diet. The ability of both fruit juices and 'baby' fruit drinks to dissolve tooth enamel is well-established (Grenby *et al.*, 1990).

'The use of sugar most closely related to rampant dental caries in infancy is the provision of fruit or fruit flavoured drinks with sugar added.'

(Rugg-Gunn, 1993)

The link between sugar-sweetened dummies and dental caries in infants has been known for some time and the COMA panel made recommendations as long ago as 1969 against the use of reservoir feeders and sweetened dummies (DHSS, 1969). Studies have since verified that there is a similar link between the use of a sweetened bottle (comforter) in infancy and infant dental caries, and that the use of a comforter is also associated with a high intake of sugar-containing snacks in later childhood.

Recommendations against the use of sweetened drinks in bottles and comforters were made in the COMA report *Dietary Sugars and Human Disease* (DoH, 1989) and this advice has been extended to include the use of fruit juices (DoH, 1994).

Practical advice about drinks

(1) Exclusively breastfed babies do not need additional fluids
(2) Give bottle fed babies cooled, boiled water in preference to all other fluids
(3) If you use baby juices:
    (a) Always follow manufacturers' instructions on usage and dilution
    (b) Serve only at mealtimes and keep drinking times short
    (c) Never use drinks on a dummy or comforter
    (d) Ideally serve from a spoon, trainer beaker or cup but not from a bottle
    (e) Do not give at bedtime or during the night

Which of the many infant drinks now available are safe for incoming teeth?

Breast milk, infant milk and cooled, boiled water are the best choices. Many 'infant' drinks contain sugars or fruit acid and are potentially harmful to teeth (cariogenic).

The following is a guide to infant drinks. Drinks for toddlers are considered in Section 23.4.

'Best choice' non-cariogenic drinks

These should constitute the majority of drinks given:

- Breast milk
- Usual infant milk
- Water (boiled and cooled until six months)

Other non-cariogenic drinks

These are safe for teeth but expensive:

- Flavoured water (if no sugars, e.g. fructose)
- 'Sugar-free' varieties of herbal drinks
- Bottled water of low mineral content (boiled and cooled until six months)

Drinks with cariogenic potential

- Dextrose or glucose water
- Any milk with added sugar
- Tea or coffee with sugar
- Flavoured follow-on milks
- 'Toddler' flavoured milk drinks
- Baby fruit juices
- 'Natural' or unsweetened fruit juices
- Baby fruit drinks or syrups
- Baby herbal drinks (except 'sugar-free' varieties)
- Flavoured water with added fructose or other sugars
- Fruit 'squash' (diluting juice)

Does 'baby' fruit juice need to be diluted?

Yes, baby juices may be less acidic than regular varieties, but still contain NME sugars. They should be well-diluted, even those purchased in ready-to-feed form. Ideally dilute until water is barely coloured, e.g. 1 tsp of juice in 100 ml of water.

What about fizzy drinks?
All carbonated drinks are unsuitable for infants as the acid content erodes dental enamel. Regular varieties are high in sugar and strongly acidic. 'Diet' varieties are acidic and contain artificial sweeteners which are banned for use in infant foods.

10.5.3 Sugars in foods

Progression through weaning on to family meals is often associated with increasing total sugar intake and frequency of intake. Extrinsic sugars are present in the diet from early weaning, in manufactured baby desserts and yoghurts, fruit purées (including home-made), some baby cereals and most rusks. Sweet biscuits and chocolate are also eaten from a young age.

The MAFF study *Nutrient Intakes of British Infants aged 6–12 months* (Mills & Tyler, 1992) found that:

- Of the 78% of all infants who ate breakfast cereal, a third had added sugar
- 63% of all infants ate cakes, buns and puddings
- 67% of infants ate biscuits
- 45% of infants ate chocolate confectionery

Why are sweet foods given to infants?
These are given for many reasons, such as rewards or treats, part of a 'natural' adaptation to a high sugar family diet, ignorance as to their potential harm to teeth, and confusion about labelling of sugars. Promotion by manufacturers of baby yoghurts and chocolate confectionery etc. encourages the purchase of sweet foods. This is a very profitable industry.

In 1985 a total of £82 million was spent advertising confectionery whilst the entire budget of the Health Education Authority in 1990/91 was £27.6 million (Rugg-Gunn, 1993).

Practical advice
It is unrealistic to expect eradication of sugar from the diet, but reducing the *frequency* of sugar intake is extremely important.

> *Frequent NME sugar intake → frequent acid production*
> *→ prolonged demineralisation = high risk of decay*

To reduce the effect of NME sugars:

- Give sweet foods at mealtimes only, and not between meals
- Do not give sweet foods before bed
- Try not to give sweet foods as rewards/sweets/bribes
- Discourage grandparents/others from giving sweet foods
- When snacks are able to be eaten, give non-sweet varieties, e.g. sandwich, bread, roll, toast, crackers, cheese scone (see Chapter 23 – Meals and Snacks)
- Brush teeth with a mild fluoride toothpaste twice per day (see Section 10.5.6)
- Be aware of the different forms of sugar

10.5.4   Sugar labelling

The following are all forms of sugar and potentially harmful to teeth:

Concentrated fruit juice

Corn syrup

Dextrose

Fruit concentrate

Fruit juice

Fruit sugar

Fructose

Glucose

Golden syrup

Honey

Invert sugar/syrup

Lactose (non-cariogenic in milk and milk products)

Malt extract

Maltodextrin

Maltose

Molasses

Raw cane sugar

Sucrose

Syrup

Treacle

10.5.5   Fluoride

Fluoride occurs naturally in drinking water, certain foods and animal and human tissues. Fluoride from the diet can enter the teeth during development and after eruption and this leads to increased resistance to demineralisation and decay. The association between the presence of fluoride in public water supplies and reduced caries has been demonstrated by over 130 surveys throughout the world. Fluoride in water at a level of 1 part per million (1 ppm) over the period of tooth development is believed to offer optimum protection against dental decay (Murray *et al.*, 1991).

Fluoridation

This is the process of 'topping up' the natural level of fluoride in water to that of 1 ppm. Some areas of England receive fluoridated water, e.g. Birmingham, Newcastle and West Cumbria, but it is not widespread.

Is water fluoridation safe?

The safety of fluoridation in respect of increased disease risk is well documented. Excess fluoride intakes can cause fluorosis (mottling of teeth) but no association has been found between fluoridation and increased risk of cancer, skeletal fluorosis or genetic damage (Knox, 1985; Freni & Gaylor, 1992). Numerous studies have failed to show any adverse effect on general health at the level of 1 ppm. Fluoride's effectiveness and safety has been endorsed by the RCP, RCGP, BDA and BMA.

Who should receive fluoride supplement?

Fluoride supplements should be used when recommended by a dentist, who will prescribe according to individual need. Supplements should *not* be given in areas where the water supply contains significant amounts of fluoride, or is fluoridated.

Supplements may be of benefit to young children at high risk of dental disease. This includes those with:

- High and frequent intakes of sugar
- Poor parental dental health
- Infrequent tooth brushing

For full protective effect, fluoride supplements need to be given daily during the period of tooth development but compliance in administering fluoride supplements is often poor.

Children thought to be at high risk should be referred to a dentist for assessment.

10.5.6 Tooth brushing

Topical application of fluoride

Fluoride can be applied topically in the form of toothpaste, and the use of fluoride toothpaste has resulted in significant caries reduction over the last 20 years. Toothpaste contains from 500 to 1500 ppm fluoride, compared to 1 ppm in fluoridated water, and therefore habitual toothpaste swallowing risks fluorosis.

Tooth brushing alone cannot prevent dental caries, but tooth brushing enables topical application of fluoride and is an effective means of plaque removal. Regular brushing to remove plaque reduces risk of periodontal (gum) disease in adolescence.

Infant tooth brushing advice for parents

- Start to brush teeth when the first tooth appears
- Brush twice per day, including last thing at night
- Use a soft 'baby' toothbrush
- Use just a tiny smear of fluoride toothpaste (size of a small pea)
- Children's toothpaste is not essential but has a milder taste and the benefit of a lower fluoride content in case of swallowing
- Try to prevent toothpaste being swallowed
- Brush your child's teeth for him/her until at least eight years of age to ensure thorough cleaning. Early established bad habits are hard to change.

10.5.7 Dental attendance

Regular dental visits should be encouraged from an early age, allowing preventive advice to be given before any damaging habits are established, familiarity with dental surroundings, pain-free visits and early detection and treatment of any problems.

What is 'an early age'?
The British Dental Health Foundation advises that infant check-ups can start from around six months. Registration with a dentist before appearance of the first tooth, and certainly by the end of the first year, is recommended. The need for attendance at such a young age is not widely understood by parents. One study found that only 28% of parents would take a child to a dentist before one year and that only 58% of health visitors advised visits before one year (Bentley, 1994).

Local policies and attitudes of dentists are known to vary. This is a likely factor contributing to confusion about the timing of first visits. Parents should be advised to ask their dentist about when they should take their infant for a first check-up. Some dentists encourage very early visits to establish familiarity with surroundings. Parents not registered with a dentist should be encouraged to do so and particular attention should be given to advice about diet and tooth brushing.

10.6   Preserving the primary dentition

Parents tend to show greater concern about conserving a child's permanent teeth (secondary dentition) than 'milk teeth' (primary dentition). This attitude is misguided.

The primary dentition preserves space in the mouth for the secondary dentition and prevents overcrowding of incoming teeth. Tooth decay causes pain and fear which in turn leads to a bad experience of the dentist. Early tooth decay requiring extraction is extremely unpleasant and risks damage to underlying teeth. Early bad dental experiences promote fear and reluctance to make later visits.

Good dental habits must be encouraged from the start because early habits are those most likely to be maintained.

10.7   Teething

Teething may encourage the use of sweetened dummies or comforter bottles and this practice must be strongly discouraged.

Practical advice

- Offer non-sweet foods, e.g. toast fingers to chew on.
- A teething ring cooled in the refrigerator may help.
- Sugar-free teething gel can be rubbed on the gums.
- 5 ml spoonful of Baby Paracetamol will relieve obvious pain.

10.8   Summary of dental health advice

- Do not use a sweetened dummy
- Give sugary foods less often and preferably only at mealtimes
- If fruit juice is given, give it well diluted and preferably only at mealtimes
- Do not give sweetened drinks from a bottle and especially for prolonged or frequent short periods of time
- Use a trainer cup from six months
- Do not give sweet drinks or foods at bedtime
- Avoid using sweets to bribe or reward
- Start tooth brushing with fluoride toothpaste as soon as a first tooth appears
- Encourage dental visits by six months

11. Food Safety

'Babies are particularly vulnerable to infection, so hygiene in preparing food takes on a new importance.'

Hull, 1992

This chapter covers:

- Factors influencing bacterial growth
- Advice on safe food storage, preparation and reheating
- Sources of common food-poisoning bacteria

Infants and young children under two years are particularly susceptible to food poisoning because their immune system is immature. Many parents are unaware of the appropriate food safety standards which should be maintained in order to minimise risk of food-borne disease. Discussion about food safety should therefore be part of advice given on feeding at all ages, from birth onwards.

11.1 Causes of food poisoning

Bacterial food poisoning is caused by either:

- Direct microbial contamination of the gut or
- The effect in the gut of toxins produced by micro-organisms

Most food has some harmful bacteria associated with it. Usually it is only when bacteria are allowed to multiply and contaminate food at high levels that there is risk of food poisoning.
   Multiplication of bacteria is influenced by:

- Temperature
- Time
- Type of food

Temperature

- *Warm temperatures* encourage bacterial growth. Growth occurs readily between 5°C and 63°C and multiplication is fastest around 37°C.

- *Refrigeration* (storage at 0–5°C) slows down the rate of multi-plication.
- *Freezing* (i.e. storage below –18°C) stops all bacterial growth but does not kill bacteria.
- *Cooking* thoroughly to a temperature of 75°C kills most bacteria.

Time

The longer food is left at a temperature conducive to multiplication of bacteria, the more prolific multiplication will be, therefore food should always be stored at temperatures which limit bacterial growth.

Type of food

Some foods are more likely to cause food poisoning than others. Bacteria need moisture to multiply and high protein foods provide ideal conditions for growth. The following 'high risk' foods must be stored and used with care:

- Cooked meat and poultry
- Eggs
- Cooked meat products
- Dairy products
- Cooked rice
- Shellfish and seafood

Bacteria do not like dry, acid or high sugar conditions. Foods such as dried infant cereal, flour, sugar, jam, biscuits etc. are 'low risk' if stored appropriately, away from moisture.

11.2   Reducing risk of food poisoning

Risk of food poisoning may be minimised if due attention is paid to:

- Kitchen hygiene
- Mealtime hygiene
- Food storage
- Food preparation

A summary of relevant points follows. See Resource List at the back of the book for sources of further information.

11.2.1   Kitchen hygiene

- Always wash hands before handling food
- Do not mix raw and cooked foods, e.g. on chopping boards; bacteria from raw foods can transfer to cooked foods
- Keep pets away when preparing foods and at mealtimes
- Clean microwave and conventional ovens regularly
- Wash dishcloths often

11.2.2   Mealtime hygiene

- Start with clean hands – both parent and child
- Clean all feeding utensils thoroughly; (sterilising is not necessary once food is eaten from a bowl)
- Sterilise bottles and teats as long as they are used
- Use a clean bib at each meal
- Serve commercial baby food from a small bowl, not from the tin or jar
- Discard food served but not eaten

11.2.3   Food storage

Unopened dried or tinned foods must be stored away from moisture, and fresh foods stored in conditions which minimise risk of bacterial growth (Table 11.1).

Refrigeration
A refrigerator (fridge) must be kept at 5°C or lower. Overloading a fridge prevents efficient circulation of cold air, and risks raising the

Table 11.1   Storage of fresh foods.

Food	Storage
Fruit, vegetables	Cool place with good ventilation or refrigerator or freezer
Milk products, eggs	Refrigerator
Meats, poultry, fish	Refrigerator, freezer
Bread	Bread bin or sealed container
Open but unserved baby meal	Refrigerator

temperature above 5°C. All refrigerated food must be covered to prevent contamination from other foods, and cooled thoroughly before storage. Uncooked foods should be stored at the bottom of the fridge to prevent dripping on to foods below.

Opened cans will rust due to the acidity of the contents, therefore food must be transferred to different containers before storage. Unserved manufactured baby foods may be kept in a fridge for up to 48 hours, but should not be reheated.

Freezing

A freezer must be kept at –18°C or lower. Only freezers which carry the three (or more) star symbol *** are capable of freezing fresh food, and those with fewer than three stars should only be used for storing ready-frozen foods, e.g. fish fingers. Foods should be frozen in good condition and cooled first if necessary.

Do not freeze:

- Half eaten jars or tins of baby food
- Food stored for some time unfrozen – it may be contaminated
- Food which has already been frozen (unless it is cooked first)

Example

> *Spaghetti bolognese sauce → defrosted → refrozen = **not safe***
> *Raw mince → defrosted → cooked to make*
> *bolognese sauce → refrozen   = safe*

11.2.4   Food preparation

Cooking

Cooking food thoroughly so that the temperature throughout the food reaches at least 75°C for two minutes kills most harmful bacteria which could cause food poisoning. Frozen food should be defrosted before cooking to prevent risk of uneven heating.

All eggs given to babies and young children must be cooked until the yolk and white are set (DoH, 1993).

Heating manufactured baby foods

Jars and tins of baby foods are sterile until open. These products can be safely heated in a basin of hot water, but should not be reheated.

Reheating food

Reheating food is a common cause of food poisoning and particular care is needed if reheating food for babies and young children. Food should be reheated until 'piping hot' (> 82°C for two minutes) and then cooled before serving; it should never be reheated more than once. Small quantities can be particularly difficult to reheat.

Safe methods for reheating small quantities:

- Heating in a covered basin over boiling water
- Heating in a small saucepan, stirring
- Heating in a covered dish in the oven
- Adding food to be reheated to another dish, and bringing to the boil, e.g. previously frozen pulses
- Microwave oven if manufacturers' instructions are observed and suitable attention is paid to heating, standing and stirring times

Note: Standing food in a basin of hot water will not reheat food to a safe temperature unless it is in sterile jars or tins.

Defrosting food

All frozen food should be thoroughly defrosted before cooking except where packaging states otherwise, e.g. frozen vegetables or fish fingers. Frozen food should be covered and thawed in the fridge and *not* in a warm environment such as a warm kitchen as this provides an ideal environment for bacteria to multiply.

A microwave oven may be used to defrost food if the food is to be eaten immediately but only the defrost/low setting (according to model) should be used for this purpose, and manufacturers' instructions for standing times must be observed. Food should be cooked or reheated and eaten as soon as possible after defrosting.

11.3 Common questions

Is it safe to cook food and store it for eating later?

Yes, provided it is cooled sufficiently to allow refrigeration or freezing within one and a half hours of cooking. Standing a bowl containing the food in iced (or very cold) water will cool it quickly. Whilst cooling, foods must be protected from contamination. Covering the container with a sheet of clean kitchen paper allows water vapour to escape and protects from airborne contamination. Food should not be covered by anything likely to cause condensation during cooling.

Food should not be cooled by putting it in the fridge (or freezer) as this will raise the fridge/freezer temperature.

Can 'baby food' be frozen?

Manufacturers do not recommend freezing their foods. Home-made foods and purées for babies can be frozen. Ice cube trays are suggested for tiny quantities and yoghurt pots for small amounts. Food must be defrosted and reheated thoroughly until piping hot.

Does cooking food in a microwave kill all harmful bacteria which could cause food poisoning?

It is the heat generated within food by the microwaves rather than the direct exposure to the microwaves which destroys bacteria. The problem with microwave ovens relates to uneven heating, resulting in hot and cold spots within the food; it is therefore essential to allow 'standing time' for the temperature throughout the food to equilibrate.

Studies have found that microwave cooking carried out in accordance with manufacturers' instructions is not wholly effective in killing listeria monocytogenes in chicken (Harrison & Carpenter, 1989). This is now thought to be attributable to the poor manufacturers' instructions at that time. Operating instructions have since been upgraded. Microwave ovens are considered to be a safe means of cooking/reheating food if instructions are followed.

Safe use of a microwave oven requires:

- Knowledge of the oven's power (wattage)
- Observation of appropriate cooking times
- Stirring food
- Observation of standing times

Microwave ovens are not recommended for heating infant milk (see Section 2.4).

Are there any 'high risk' foods which should not be given to infants and young children?

The following foods should not be given to infants and young children under two years of age:

- Raw or lightly cooked eggs (DoH, 1993)
- Foods made with uncooked eggs, e.g. mousse, ice cream, mayonnaise (DoH, 1993)

- Unpasteurised milk, including goat and ewe (DoH, 1994)
- Unpasteurised cheese
- Soft or blue-veined cheeses e.g. brie, camembert, Danish blue
- Paté
- Pre-cooked poultry
- Shellfish
- Soft whip ice cream from machines

11.4   Common food poisoning bacteria

There are many groups of food poisoning bacteria. The most common and well recognised are salmonella, listeria, campylobacter, staphylococcus, Escherichia coli.

11.4.1   Salmonella

Symptoms – Diarrhoea, abdominal pain, vomiting; starts 12–24 hours after eating. Can be fatal in the very young.
Found in – Unpasteurised milk, eggs, poultry, meat, left-over food.

Advice to reduce risk

- Avoid raw or lightly cooked eggs or dishes containing them, e.g. soft scrambled egg, home-made mayonnaise, ice cream.
- Salmonella bacteria are killed by high temperatures. Cook meat and poultry thoroughly (to 75°C). Cook eggs until yolk and white are *solid*.
- Avoid cross contamination from raw to cooked foods (see Section 11.2.1).
- Ensure adequate defrosting of meat and poultry.
- Do not use cracked eggs.

11.4.2   Listeria

Found widely distributed in the environment, i.e. soil, vegetation, and animals.
Dangerous – because it can thrive at temperatures as low as 3°C and can survive microwave cooking even when instructions are followed.
Symptoms – Flu-like symptoms starting 5–30 days after eating.
Especially dangerous in infants – can be fatal.
Found in – soft ripened cheeses e.g. brie, camembert (including those

made from pasteurised milk), paté, ice cream (especially soft whip variety from machines).

Advice to reduce risk

- Avoid giving high risk foods before two years (see Section 11.3).
- Re-heat cook–chill meals and ready-to-eat poultry > 75°C
- Avoid all unpasteurised milk and milk products, e.g. goat's milk
- Wash all fruit and vegetables thoroughly in running water

11.4.3 Campylobacter

The infective dose for this illness is low since no multiplication of the bacteria on food is required and direct hand to mouth infection is common.

Animals such as cats, dogs and sheep may be host to campylobacter. Young children may transfer bacteria to their mouths by playing near infected animals. Campylobacter is thought to be a major source of gastroenteritis in young children.

Found in – Unpasteurised milk, meat, poultry.

Advice to reduce risk

- Encourage good personal hygiene, i.e. wash hands before handling food.
- Keep pets away from work surfaces and cooking utensils.
- Avoid cross contamination from raw to cooked foods.
- Avoid unpasteurised milk products.

11.4.4 Staphylococcus

The causative agent in relation to this bacteria is an exotoxin (heat resistant toxin which can survive boiling for 30 minutes or 121°C for 11 minutes, i.e. pressure cooking). The organism itself is destroyed by heating to 70°C but the toxin is still viable.

The skin of the hands and the nose often harbours staphylococci. Contamination of food follows from contact with unwashed hands or from sneezing.

Symptoms – Vomiting and stomach cramps start 1–6 hours after eating.

Found in – Food that needs handling, e.g. sandwiches, salads, meat and poultry eaten cold; cold desserts, e.g. custard, trifle.

Advice to reduce risk

- Cover all cuts on hands
- Wash hands thoroughly before handling food
- Avoid coughing or sneezing over food
- Cover prepared foods

11.4.5 Escherichia coli

Escherichia coli is a natural inhabitant of both animal and human gut without causing any illness. There are, however, strains of this bacteria which are capable of producing toxins which can lead to serious illness such as E. coli 0157.

The main source of the bacteria is almost certainly cattle but it can be spread in a number of ways. The infective dose is very small and there have been a few cases where direct contact with cattle or humans has caused illness.

The illness may be particularly severe in the elderly and young who are most at risk, and in a number of cases infection will lead to hospitalisation.

Symptoms – These range from mild diarrhoea to bloody and severe diarrhoea and abdominal pain which can lead to renal failure and anaemia. The symptoms present 2–8 days after infection, although 14 day incubation periods are not uncommon.

Found in – Raw meats, unpasteurised milk, cheeses made with unpasteurised milk. E. coli 0157 has been associated with food poisoning outbreaks following consumption of unpasteurised cheese, milk where the pasteurisation process failed and undercooked burgers; recently cooked meats have also been implicated, indicating precautions must be taken to prevent cross contamination from raw to cooked foods.

Advice to reduce risks
Wash all vegetables thoroughly; use of cattle manure as a 'natural fertiliser' has been linked to outbreaks.

Public water supplies treatment is effective against this organism. Care must be taken to boil any water used from streams etc., particularly in areas where farm animals are grazed.

11.4.6 Rotavirus infection

Rotavirus infection is common in infants and young children, but it is rarely food related.

11.5 Summary   10%

Infants and young children are considered to be at greater risk from poisoning than older children and adults. Risks can be minimised by awareness of common-sense principles of storing and preparing foods. Avoidance of 'high risk' foods is advised for the first two years. Particular care should be taken with reheating foods.

References and Further Reading for Section 1

Adler, B.R. & Warner, J.O. (1991) Food intolerance in children. In *Royal College of General Practitioners Members Reference Book* pp. 497–502 RCGP, London.

American Academy of Pediatrics: Commission on Nutrition (1986) Aluminium toxicity in infants and children. *Pediatrics*, 78, 1150–54.

American Academy of Pediatrics: Committee on Nutrition (1992) The use of whole cow's milk in infancy. *Pediatrics*, 89, 1105–9.

Anyon, C.P. & Clarkson, K.G. (1969) Occult gastrointestinal bleeding in the first two months of life. *New Zealand Medical Journal*, 70, 316–17.

Barker, D.J.P., Winter, P.D., Osmond, C., Margetts, B. & Simmonds, S.J. (1989) Weight in infancy and death from ischaemic heart disease. *Lancet*, 2, 577–80.

Beeken, S. & Waterston, T. (1992) Health Service support of breast-feeding – are we practising what we preach? *B.M.J.*, 305, 285–87.

Bentley, E. (1994) Views about preventive dental care for infants. *Health Visitor*, March, 67, (3).

Bergevin Y. Dougherty, C. & Kramer, M.S. (1983) Do infant formula samples shorten breast-feeding? *Lancet*, i, 1148–51.

Billeaud, C., Guillet, J. & Sandler, B. (1990) Gastric emptying in infants with or without gastro-oesophageal reflux according to the type of milk. *European J. of Clin. Nutr.*, 44, 577–83.

Bloom, K., Goldbloom, R., Robinson, S. & Stevens, F. (1982) Factors affecting the continuance of breast-feeding. *Acta. Ped. Scand.*, 300 (Suppl), 9–14.

Bock, S., May C.D. & Remigio, L. (1979) *The Mast Cell: its Role in Health and Disease* (J. Pepys & A.M. Edwards). Pitman Medical, Tunbridge Wells.

Broadbent, J.B. & Sampson, H.A. (1988) Food hypersensitivity and atopic dermatitis. *Paediatric Allergic Disease*, 35, 1115.

Campbell, H. & Jones, I.G. (1994) Scottish needs assessment programme. *Health Promotion Review. Breast-feeding in Scotland.*

Cant, A.J. (1991) Early diet and later allergic disease. *British Nutrition Foundation Bulletin*, June, 16, Suppl.1, 52–73.

Cant, A.J. & Bailes, J.A. (1984) How should we feed the potentially allergic infant? *Human Nutr.: Appl. Nutr.*, 38A, 474–76.

Cant, A.J., Bailes, J.A., Marsden, R.A. & Hewitt, D. (1986) Effect of maternal dietary exclusion on breast-fed infants with eczema: two controlled studies. *B.M.J.*, 293, 231–3.

Carter, C. (1994) The Immune System. In *Clinical Paediatric Dietetics* (eds Shaw & Lawson). Blackwell Science Ltd, Oxford.

de Carvalho, M., Hall, M. & Harvey D. (1981) Effect of water supplementation on physiological jaundice in breast-fed babies. *Arch. Dis. Child*, **56** (7) 568–9.

de Carvalho, M., Robertson, S., Friedman, A. & Klaus, M. (1982) Effect of frequent breastfeeding on early milk production and infant weight gain. *Paediatrics*, **72** (3) 307–11.

Chan, G.M., McMurry, M., Westover, K., Englebert-Fenton, K. & Thomas, M.R. (1987) Effects of increased dietary calcium intake upon calcium and bone mineral status in lactating adolescent and adult women. *Am. J. Clin. Nutr.*, **46**, 319–23.

Chandra, R.K., Puri, S. & Hamed, A. (1989) Influence of maternal diet during lactation and use of formula feeds on development of atopic eczema in high risk infants. *BMJ*, **299**, 228–30.

Cushing, A. & Gelbier, S. (1988) The dental health of children attending day nurseries in three inner London boroughs. *J. Pediatric Dent.*, **4**, 77–85.

David, T.J. (1993) *Food and Food Additive Intolerance in Childhood*. Blackwell Science Ltd, Oxford.

DHSS (1969) Department of Health & Social Security panel on cariogenic foods. Committee on Medical Aspects of Food Policy (COMA). First Report, *Br. Dent. J.*, **126**, 273–7.

DHSS (1977) Department of Health & Social Security. The Composition of Mature Human Milk. *Report on Health and Social Subjects* No. 12. HMSO, London.

DHSS (1980) Department of Health & Social Security. Artificial Feeds for the Young Infant. *Report on Health and Social Subjects No. 18*. HMSO, London.

DHSS (1988a) Department of Health & Social Security. Present Day Practice in Infant Feeding. Third Report. *Report on Health and Social Subjects No. 32*. HMSO, London.

DHSS (1988b) Department of Health & Social Security. *HIV Infection, Breast-feeding and Human Milk Banking*. PL/CMO 13. HMSO, London.

DoH (1989) Dietary Sugars and Human Disease. *Report on Health and Social Subjects No. 37*. HMSO, London.

DoH (1991) Department of Health Dietary Reference Values for Food, Energy and Nutrients for the United Kingdom. Report of the Panel on Dietary Reference Values of the Committee on Medical Aspects of Food Policy. *Report on Health and Social Subjects No. 41*. HMSO, London.

DoH (1993) Department of Health. Advisory committee on the microbiological safety of food. *Report on Salmonella in Eggs*. HMSO, London.

DoH (1994) Department of Health. Weaning and the Weaning Diet (COMA). *Report on Health and Social Subjects No. 45*. HMSO, London.

DoH (1995) Department of Health. *Infant Formula and Follow-on Formula Regulations.* SI No. 77. HMSO, London.

Dusdieker, L.B., Booth, B.M., Stumbo, P.J. & Eichenberger, J.M. (1985) Effect of supplementary fluids on human milk production. *J. of Paediatrics,* **106,** 207–11.

Edwards, A.G.K., Halse, P.C., Parkin, J.M. & Waterston, A.J.R. (1990) Recognising failure to thrive in early childhood. *Arch. Dis. Child.,* **65,** 1263–5.

Erhardt, P. (1986) Iron deficiency in young Bradford children from different ethnic groups. *B.M.J.,* **292,** 90–93.

ESPGAN (1987) European Society of Paediatric Gastroenterology and Nutrition. Nutrition and feeding of preterm infants. *Acta. Ped. Scand.,* Suppl. 536.

Farquharson, J., Cockburn, F. Patrick, A.W., Janneson, E.C. & Logan, R.W. (1992) Infant cerebral cortex phospholipid fatty-acid composition and diet. *B.M.J.,* **306,** 810.

Fergusson, D.M., Horwood, L.J. & Shannon, F.T. (1990) Early solid feeding and recurrent childhood eczema: a 10 year longitudinal study. *Pediatrics,* **86,** 541–6.

FMF (1983) *Code of Practice for Marketing of Infant Formulae in the United Kingdom and Schedule for a Code Monitoring Committee.* Food Manufacturers' Federation, London.

Forsyth, S.J., Ogston, S.A., Clark, A., Florey, C. du V. & Howie, P.W. (1993) Relation between early introduction of solid food to infants and their weight and illness during the first two years of life. *B.M.J.,* **306,** 1572–6.

Frankl, D.A. & Zeisel, S.H. (1988) Failure to Thrive. *The Paediatric Clinics of N. America,* **35,** 6, December.

Freeman, J.V., Cole, T.J., Chinn, S., Jones, P.R., White, E.M. & Preece, M.A. (1995) Cross sectional stature and weight reference curves for the UK, 1990. *Arch. Dis. Child,* **73,** 17–24.

Freni, S.C. & Gaylor, D.W. (1992) International trends in the incidence of bone cancer are not related to drinking water fluoridation. *Cancer,* **70,** 611–18.

Goldberg, N.M. & Adams, E. (1983) Supplementary water for breast-fed babies in a hot, dry climate. Not really a necessity. *Arch. Dis. Child.,* January, 73–4.

Gray-Donald K., Kramer, M.S., Munday, S. & Leduc, D.G. (1985) Effect of formula supplementation in hospital on the duration of breast-feeding: a controlled trial. *Pediatrics,* **75** (3) 514–18.

Greer F.R., Ho, M., Dodson, D. & Tsang R.C. (1981) Lack of 25-hydroxyvitamin D and 1,25–dihydroxyvitamin D in human milk. *J. Pediat,* **99,** 233–5.

Gregory, J.R., Collins, D.L. Davies P.S.W., Clark, P.C. & Hughes, J.M. (1995) *National Diet and Nutrition Survey of Children Aged $1\frac{1}{2}$ and $4\frac{1}{2}$ years.* HMSO, London.

Grenby, T.H., Mistry, M. & Desai, T. (1990) Potential dental effects of infants' fruit drinks studied *in vivo*. *Br. J. Nutr*, **64**, 273–83.

Hales, C.N., Barker, D.J.P., Clark, P.M.S., Cox, L.J., Fall, C. & Osmond, C. (1991) Fetal and infant growth and impaired glucose tolerance at age 64. *B.M.J.*, **303**, 1019–22.

Harrison, M.A. & Carpenter, S.L. (1989) Survival of Listeria Monocytogenes in microwave-cooked poultry. *Food Microbiology*, **6**, 153–7.

HEA (1992) *A Handbook of Dental Health for Health Visitors*. Health Education Board, London.

HEA (1994) *The National Food Guide. The Balance of Good Health*. Health Education Board, London.

HEA (1996) *The Scientific Basis of Dental Health Education*. A policy document, 4th ed. Health Education Board, London.

Hernell, O. (1990) The requirements and utilisation of dietary fatty acids in the newborn infant. *Acta.Paediatr.Scand*. Suppl. 365, 20–27.

Hindmarsh, P.C. & Brook, C.G.D. (1986) Measuring the growth of children in general practice. *Maternal & Child Health*, June.

HMSO (1995) The Infant Formula and Follow-on Formula Regulations 1995. SI 1995 No. 77. HMSO, London.

Holt, R.D. (1990). Caries in the pre-school child: British trends. *J. Dent.*, **18**, 196–299.

Howard, F.M., Howard C.R. & Weitzman, M. (1993) The physician as advertiser: the unintentional discourgement of breast-feeding. *Obstetrics & Gynaecology*, **81** (b), 1048–51.

Howie, P.W., Forsyth, J.S., Ogston, S.A., Clark, A. & Florey C. du V. (1990) Protective effect of breastfeeding against infection. *B.M.J.*, **300**, 11–16.

Hyde, L. (1994) Knowledge of basic infant nutrition amongst community health professionals. *Maternal and Child Health*. January, 27–32.

Idjradinata P., Watkins, W.E. & Pollitt, E. (1993) Adverse effect of iron supplementation on weight gain of iron replete young children. *Lancet*, **343**, 1252–4.

Illingworth, R.S. (1964) The critical or sensitive period with special reference to certain feeding problems in infants and children. *J. Pediat*, **65**, 839–49.

Illingworth, P.J., Jung, R.T., Howie, P.W., Leslie, P. & Isles, T.E. (1986) Diminution in energy expenditure during lactation. *B.M.J.*, **292**, 437–41.

Kitchen, W.H., Ford, G.W. & Doyle, L.W. (1989) Growth and very low birth weight. *Arch. Dis. Child.*, **64**, 379–82.

Kjellman, N-IM. (1977) Atopic disease in seven year old children. *Acta. Paediatr. Scand.*, **66**, 456–71.

Knox, E.G. (1985) *Fluoridation of Water and Cancer: A Review of the Epidemiological Evidence*. HMSO, London.

Lawson, M. (1991) Low birthweight infants. In *Clinical Paediatric Dietetics* Shaw V. & Lawson M. (eds). Blackwell Science Ltd., Oxford.

Lucas, A. (1994) Feeding the normal infant. *Medicine International*, 22 (10) 396–401.

Lucas, A. & Cole, T.J. (1990) Breast milk and neonatal necrotising enterocolitis. *Lancet*, 336, 1519–23.

Lucas, A., Ewing, G., Roberts, S.B. & Coward, W.A. (1987) How much energy does the breast-fed infant consume and expend? *B.M.J.*, 295, 75–7.

Lucas, A., Morley, A., Cole, T.J., Gore, S.M., Davis, J.A., Bamford, M.F. & Dossetor J.F. (1989) Early diet in preterm babies and developmental status in infancy. *Arch. Dis. Child.*, 64, 1570–78.

Lucas, A., Morley, R., Coles, T.J., Lister, G. & Leeson-Payne, C. (1992a) Breast milk and subsequent intelligence quotient in children born preterm. *Lancet*, 340, 261–4.

Lucas, A., Bishop, N.J., King, F.J. & Cole, T.J. (1992b) Randomised trial of nutrition for preterm infants after discharge. *Arch. Dis. Child.*, 67, 324–7.

Marcovitch, H. (1994) Failure to thrive. *B.M.J.* 308, 1 January.

Marder, A., Nicoll, A., Polnay, L. & Shulman, C.E. (1990) Discovering anaemia at child health clinics. *Arch. Dis. Child.*, 65, 892–4.

Milla, P.J. (1988) Intestinal absorption and digestion of nutrients. In *Fetal and Neonatal Growth* (ed. F. Cockburn) pp.93–103, John Wiley, Chichester.

Mills, A.F. (1990) Surveillance for anaemia: risk factors in patterns of milk intake. *Arch. Dis. Child.*, 65, 428–31.

Mills A. & Tyler, H. (1992) *Food and Nutrient Intakes of British Infants aged 6–12 months*. HMSO, London.

Miskelly, F.G., Burr, M.L., Vaughan-Williams, E., Fehily, A.M., Butland, B.K. & Merrett, T.G. (1988) Infant feeding and allergy. *Arch.Dis.Child.*, 63, 388–93.

Morgan, J.B., Redfern, A.M. & Stordy, B.J. (1993) Nutritional composition (by chemical analysis) of home prepared weaning foods for infants. *Proc. Nutr. Soc. (International Proceedings Abstracts)*, 21–23 Sept.

Morse, E. (1988). *My Child Won't Eat*. Penguin, London.

Moynihan, P.J., Wright, W.G. & Walton, A.G. (1996) A comparison of the relative acidogenic potential of infant milk and soya infant formula: a plaque pH study. *Int. J. of Paediatric Dentristry*, 6, 177–81.

Murray, J.J., Breckon, J.A., Reynolds, P.J., Tabari, E.D. & Nunn, J.H. (1991) The effect of residence and social class on dental caries experience in 15–16 year old children living in three towns in the North East of England. *Br.Dent.J*, 171, 319–22.

Neu, J., Valentine, C. & Meetze, W. (1990) Scientifically based strategies for nutrition of the high risk, low birthweight infant. *European J.Paediatr.*, 150, 2–13.

Newcomb, P.A., Storer, B.E., Longnecker, M.P., Mittendorf, R., Greenberg, E.R., Clapp, R.W., Burke, K.P., Willett, W.C. & MacMahon, B. (1994) Lactation and a reduced risk of premenopausal breast cancer. *New Eng.J.Med.*, 330(2) 81–7.

RCM (1991) *Successful Breastfeeding*, 2nd ed. Royal College of Midwives/ Churchill Livingstone, Edinburgh

RCP/BNF (1984) Joint Report of the Royal College of Physicians and the British Nutrition Foundation. Food Intolerance and Food Aversion. M.H. Lessof, (chairman). *J. Royal Coll. Phys.*, 18(2) 83–134.

Roper, N. (ed) (1980) *Churchill Livingstone Pocket Medical Dictionary*, 13th edn. Churchill Livingstone, Edinburgh.

Rugg-Gunn, A.J. (1993) *Nutrition and Dental Health*. Oxford Medical Publications, Oxford.

Salariya, E.M., Easton, P.M. & Carter, J.I. (1978) Duration of feeding after early initiation and frequent feeding. *Lancet*, ii, 1141–3.

Skuse, D. (1992) Failure to thrive: current perspectives. *Current Paediatr.*, 105–10.

Skuse, D. (1993) Identification and management of problem eaters. *Arch. Dis. Child.*, **69**, 604–8.

Smith, D. (1995) *Baby Food Watch*. Harper Collins, London.

SODH/CMO (1996) Scottish Office Department of Health/Chief Medical Officer. *Letter and Patient Information Sheet 18*, 17 July 1996.

Stordy, B.J. *et al.* (1993) Nutritional composition (by chemical analysis) of sweet home prepared weaning foods for infants. 1. Energy and macro-nutrients. *Proc. Nutr. Soc. (International Proceedings Abstracts)* 21–23 Sept.

Taitz, L.S. & Scholey, E. (1989) Are babies more satisfied by casein based formulas? *Arch.Dis.Child.*, **64**, 619–21.

Taitz, L.S. & Wardley, B.L. (1990) *Handbook of Child Nutrition*. Oxford University Press, Oxford.

Tanner, J.M., Whitehouse, R. H. & Takaishi, M. (1966) Standards from birth to maturity for height, weight, height velocity and weight velocity in British children. *Arch.Dis.Child.*, **41**, 454–72 (Part I); 613–25 (Part II).

Thomas, B. (ed) (1994) *Manual of Dietetic Practice*, 2nd edn. Blackwell Science Ltd, Oxford.

Toumba, K.J. & Curzon, M.E.J. (1994) The fluoride content of bottled waters. *Br.Dent.J*, **176**, 266–8.

Trounce, J.Q. & Walker-Smith, J.A. (1985) Sugar intolerance complicating acute gastroenteritis. *Arch.Dis.Child*, **60**, 986–90

Uauy, R., Birch, E., Birch, D. & Peirano, P. (1992) Visual and brain function measurements in studies in n-3 fatty acid requirements of infants. *J.Pediatr*, **120**, S168–80.

Wharton, B. (1990) Milk for babies and children. *B.M.J.*, **301**, 774–5.

White, A., Freeth, S. & O'Brien, M. (1992) *Infant Feeding 1990*. OPCS, HMSO, London.

WHO (1972) Nutritional Anaemias. *World Health Organisation Technical Report Series, No. 503*. WHO, Geneva.

WHO (1992) *Global Program on AIDS*. Consensus statement from the

WHO/UNICEF consultation on HIV transmission and breast-feeding. 30 April–1 May, 1992, Geneva. World Health Organisation GPAINF 92.1

WHO/UNICEF (1981) *International Code of Marketing of Breast Milk Substitutes*. World Health Organisation, Geneva.

WHO/UNICEF (1989) *Joint statement: Protecting, Promoting and Supporting Breast-feeding: the Special Role of Maternity Services*. WHO, Geneva.

Woodruff, C. W., Latham, C. & McDavid, S. (1977) Iron nutrition in the breast-fed infant. *J. of Pediatrics*, **90**, 36–8.

Woolridge, M. & Fisher, C. (1988) Colic, 'overfeeding' and symptoms of lactose malabsorption in the breast-fed baby: a possible artefact of feed management? *Lancet.* **2**, 382–4.

Further reading

CEC (1991) Commission of the European Communities. Directive on infant formulae and follow-on formulae. 91/321/EEC. *Off. J. Eur. Commun*, L175, 35–49.

Hull, S. (1992) *Safe Cooking for a Healthy Baby*. Penguin, London.

Lönnerdal, B. (1994) Nutritional aspects of soy formula. *Acta. Paediatr. Suppl.*, **402**, 105–108.

Porter, B. & Skuse, D. (1991) When does slow weight gain become failure to thrive? *Arch. Dis. Child.*, **66**, 905–6.

Shaw, V. & Lawson, M. (eds.) (1994) *Clinical Paediatric Dietetics*. Blackwell Science Ltd, Oxford.

Walker-Smith, J. (1987) Commentary on gastrointestinal food allergy in childhood. In *Food Intolerance* (ed. J. Dobbing). Baillière Tindall, London.

Zoppi, G., Gasparini, R., Mantovanelli, F. Gobio-Casali, L., Astolfi, R. & Crovari, P. (1983) Diet and antibody response to vaccination in health infants. *Lancet*, **ii**, 11–14.

Section 2
One to Three Years

12. Nutritional Requirements 1–3 Years

> 'Infants and children are not mini adults; they require different nutrients and a different balance of nutrients.'
>
> Stordy, 1994

The term 'toddler' is used to describe a child aged 1–3 years of age. This chapter covers:

- The differences between toddler and adult nutrient needs
- Practical advice about how nutrient needs can be met

12.1 Introduction

The years from one to three are a stage of dietary transition from infant to adult-style eating when two dietary goals can be identified:

(1) To achieve dietary adequacy in respect of all nutrients so as to enable optimal growth and development
(2) To encourage 'healthy eating habits' with a view to minimising later risk of diet-related diseases

Balancing these two goals can be difficult.

12.2 Nutrient needs

The diet of any young child must provide adequate energy and nutrients for:

- Growth
- Building body nutrient stores
- Body maintenance and repair
- Day to day activities

Although rate of growth from 1–3 years is less than in infancy, nutrient needs are still high in relation to body size (see Table 12.1). Toddlers

Table 12.1 Estimated average requirements of energy for males.

Age	Energy kcal/kg body weight/day
Neonates	115
At 12 months	95
At 3 years	95
At 5 years	88
At 18 years	43
Adult	34

From: DoH, 1991 (abridged from Table 2: Energy).

have a small stomach capacity and often variable appetites. They therefore require a nutrient-dense diet to enable energy and nutrient needs to be met. The period from 1–5 years is particularly important for brain and functional development. A poor diet providing either insufficient energy or an insufficient amount of specific nutrients can have an adverse effect on both growth and development.

A diet considered healthy for adults, which is low in fat and high in fibre, is not suitable for young children because of its low energy density and high bulk. Limited adoption of healthy eating guidelines can be encouraged from two years (see Chapter 14), but it is important to remember that young children are not small adults and the need for dietary adequacy in respect of all nutrients is of paramount importance.

What is a healthy diet for toddlers?
A healthy diet should provide sufficient nutrients in appropriate proportions to enable optimal growth and development, i.e. a balance of:

- Protein
- Carbohydrate
- Fat
- Fibre
- Vitamins
- Minerals
- Water

How can this be achieved?

Different foods supply different combinations of nutrients and certain types of food tend to be good sources of specific nutrients. A balanced intake of nutrients is most readily achieved by eating a variety of different foods. The ideal healthy diet for toddlers is therefore a varied diet. This is discussed further in Chapter 6 – Weaning and Section 12.4.

12.3 Dietary reference values

The nutrient needs of young children were reviewed by the Committee on Medical Aspects of Food Policy (COMA) Panel on Dietary Reference Values set up in 1987 and described in the 1991 report of the Panel (DoH, 1991). Dietary Reference Values (DRVs) is a term which covers all figures produced by the Panel including:

- *Estimated Average Requirements (EAR)* – average requirement for food energy or a nutrient
- *Reference Nutrient Intake (RNI)* – amount of a nutrient that is enough for almost every individual, even someone who has high needs for the nutrient.

Young children show considerable variation in their individual nutrient requirements. This is attributable to differences in:

- Sex
- Weight
- Height
- Age
- Requirements for growth
- Body stores of nutrients
- Activity level
- Genetic factors

DRVs must therefore be used as an indication and not a definition of a child's requirements for any given nutrient. DRVs for children aged 1–3 years are given in Appendix II.

How much energy is required?

Energy requirements must be met to enable satisfactory growth, and toddler energy requirements are high in relation to body weight (see Table 12.2). Male and female average energy requirements per

Table 12.2   Estimated average energy requirements at 50th centile weight.

Age	Energy kcal/day (male)	Energy kcal/day (female)
1 year	960	910
2 years	1190	1130
3 years	1380	1320

From: DoH, 1991, Table 2.1.

kilogram of body weight are the same from 12 months to 3 years (i.e. 95 kcals/kg/day). Male requirements are greater than female requirements at any given age because their lean body mass is greater.

What about other nutrient requirements at this age?
Requirements are detailed in Appendix II.

Protein
1.1 g protein per kg body weight per day is needed to maintain tissue growth. Adequate energy intake is essential otherwise protein is metabolised as energy. Foods from the meat, fish and alternatives food group are rich in protein, although significant amounts are also supplied from foods in other groups, e.g. milk.

Calcium
A daily intake of 350 mg calcium is required to maintain healthy bone development. Approximately 250 mg calcium is provided from each of the following:

- 180 ml ($\frac{1}{3}$ pint) whole or semi-skimmed milk
- 150 g (5 oz) carton of yoghurt
- 35 g ($1\frac{1}{4}$ oz) cheddar-type cheese
- 60 g (2 oz) sardines or other soft-boned fish

Approximately 125 mg calcium is provided from:

- 100 ml ($\frac{1}{6}$ pint) whole or semi-skimmed milk
- Two cheese spread triangles
- Two scoops of non-dairy ice cream
- 100 g ($\frac{1}{6}$ pint) milk pudding
- 4×40 g ($1\frac{1}{2}$ oz) pots of fromage frais

Vitamin D
Vitamin D deficiency may lead to poor bone mineralisation (rickets). A daily intake of 7 µg vitamin D is recommended but dietary sources are limited and skin synthesis of vitamin D is restricted in winter. Supplements are therefore recommended for children aged 1–3 years (DoH, 1991; DoH, 1994).

Iron
A daily intake of 6.9 mg is advocated. Toddlers commonly have low iron stores. Iron status can be optimised by daily consumption of iron-rich foods and a good intake of vitamin C rich foods.

Zinc
Zinc is required for good growth and weight gain and deficiency may be seen in cases of failure to thrive. Zinc is obtained from foods in the meat, fish and alternatives and milk and dairy foods groups.

Vitamin C
A daily supply of vitamin C is required because large amounts cannot be stored in the body. Vitamin C plays an important role in enhancing iron absorption.

Dietary fibre (non-starch polysaccharide)
There is no DRV for fibre for young children. A moderate fibre intake is desirable (see Section 14.2), but high fibre foods must not be given at the expense of energy-rich foods.

12.4   Meeting nutrient needs

Parents need practical advice about how to ensure toddler nutrient needs are met. A varied diet should be strongly encouraged to ensure the availability of a wide range of nutrients (see Section 12.2) and the idea of appropriate dietary variety should be explained with reference to the following food groups:

- Milk and dairy foods
- Meat, fish and alternatives
- Bread, other cereals and potatoes
- Fruit and vegetables

Fatty and sugary foods are considered to be dietary 'extras' because they are of low nutritional value, e.g. cakes, sweets, crisps and sweet drinks. However, some fatty foods, e.g. butter, margarine and oils, do provide important vitamins and fatty acids.

How big is a serving?

It is not particularly practical to define serving sizes for all groups since they will vary considerably throughout childhood. Serving size should be determined according to appetite and can be considered as any portion larger than 1–2 mouthfuls. Exceptionally, one serving of milk (from the milk and dairy foods group) is generally regarded to be 180 ml ($\frac{1}{3}$ pint) of milk or equivalent (see Section 12.3). However, three or four smaller servings per day are often more practical for toddlers.

How many choices should be made from each group?

The number of daily servings advised is shown in Table 12.3.

Table 12.3 Recommended number of daily servings.

Food group	Minimum servings per day
Milk and dairy foods	2–3
Meat, fish and alternatives	2 small
Bread, other cereals and potatoes	4 or more, depending on appetite
Fruit and vegetables 　　Fruit 　　Vegetables	1–2 1–2
Fatty and sugary foods	Moderate amount of butter or margarine Limited other choices Limit sweet drinks to meal times

13. Assessing Dietary Adequacy

> 'The assessment of childhood diet is both an important and emotive issue.'
>
> Davies & Evans, 1995

This chapter covers:

- Major risk factors for dietary inadequacy
- Obtaining a 24 hour diet history
- Assessment of dietary adequacy using the food groups

Normal child growth and development is dependent on nutrient needs being met. It is often assumed that toddlers do receive an overall 'adequate' diet, but there are many reasons why this may not be so. Nutritional inadequacy may be the result of:

- An inadequate energy intake
- Lack of variety in the diet
- An inadequate intake of foods rich in specific nutrients
- All of the above

Given the long-term consequences of undernutrition, monitoring of dietary adequacy is very important. Community health professionals are well placed to identify toddlers at risk of nutritional inadequacy, enabling early intervention before the onset of growth failure. Referral must be made to a dietitian whenever a child is considered to be at nutritional risk, or if a detailed nutritional assessment is required.

Four tiers of assessment can be defined:

(1) Risk factors for dietary inadequacy, i.e. identification of the toddler at risk
(2) Growth and wellbeing
(3) Dietary composition and range of different foods eaten
(4) Dietary provision of individual nutrients

13.1 Risk factors for dietary inadequacy

A number of factors may increase the risk of a young child failing to achieve an adequate nutritional intake. It must be noted, however, that risk of dietary inadequacy does not necessarily result in dietary inadequacy.

13.1.1 Social

- Low income (NCH, 1991)
- Lack of knowledge of child nutrition
- Lack of cooking facilities
- Irregular family meals
- Poor parent–child interaction (Casey et al., 1984)
- Working mother

13.1.2 Cultural

- Asian family (Warrington & Storey, 1988)
- Afro-Caribbean family
- Rastafarian family

13.1.3 Dietary

- Special dietary requirements, e.g. gluten free, milk free
- Inappropriate dietary restriction or exclusion
- Vegan diet
- Macrobiotic diet
- Vegetarian diet
- Inappropriate family diet
- Prolonged food refusal
- Excessive and prolonged food faddiness
- Excessive fluid intake (Hourihane & Rolles, 1995)
- High intake of sweets ('extras')
- Over zealous application of adult healthy eating guidelines
- Early weaning
- Inappropriate weaning diet

13.1.4 Medical

Malabsorption   cystic fibrosis
                              bowel resection
                              coeliac disease
                              acute gastrointestinal infection

Inadequate intake/	chronic illness, e.g. asthma
increased requirement	cardiac problems
	respiratory problems
	recurrent infection
	feeding difficulties

13.2   Growth and wellbeing

Assessment of growth is a central part of any assessment of nutritional status and dietary adequacy. Measurement of weight, height and head circumference should be made for any child whose diet is giving cause for concern and the results should be plotted on centile charts for longitudinal comparison. If growth is satisfactory, energy and protein intake is likely to be adequate. However, growth adequacy does not imply dietary adequacy in respect of all nutrients. Specific nutrient intake, e.g. iron, may be sub-optimal. If this is suspected, check dietary variety (see next sections).

Assessment of child wellbeing should be made in association with anthropometric assessment of growth. This provides a means of identifying the possible duration, cause and potential significance of any nutritional problem. The following action is suggested:

Any toddler who appears unwell, or continues to show poor weight gain, should be referred for medical and dietetic assessment.

13.3   Dietary composition

The food groups provide a straightforward means of assessing the dietary variety and hence nutritional balance of a toddler's diet. The 'ideal' toddler diet can be described in terms of daily servings from each of the food groups. Comparison of an individual toddler's diet with the 'ideal' then gives a guide to its adequacy.

Obtaining a 24 hour diet history is the first step in assessing toddler dietary composition and variety.

13.3.1   The diet history

The diet history is a retrospective record of everything consumed by an individual in a given period. The idea is simple, but it can be difficult to achieve in practice.

Eight steps to a meaningful diet history

(1) Explain to the parent(s) what information you are looking for, i.e. a description of what the toddler eats and drinks in a typical 24 hour period.

(2) Ask them to think about what the toddler ate yesterday. It is much easier to focus on a single day.

(3) Start from waking and ask about food and drink taken through the day as follows:

- waking
- breakfast
- mid-morning
- lunch
- mid-afternoon
- early evening meal
- late evening
- before bed

(4) Memories are notoriously deceptive and individuals' perceptions of eating episodes differ, so it is important to backtrack and ask about food and drink consumption in different ways. Parents' anxiety about a child's refusal to eat may, in addition, cause them to overlook the small amounts that are eaten. Backtracking questions might include:

- 'Does he like sweets/chocolate/biscuits? When might he eat them?'
- 'What is the next thing he would have to eat?' This avoids any confusion about perceptions of meals and mealtimes.
- 'What drinks does he like? When does he have a drink?'

(5) Approximate quantities can be helpful, e.g. $\frac{1}{2}$ cup or three cups of milk. However, don't be too concerned about quantities eaten/drunk. Appetites vary greatly. The frequency with which a food is eaten is more important.

(6) Record only food *eaten*, not food *offered*. This can make a big difference to a day's intake. Remember to include the 'two mouthfuls' of carrots etc.

(7) Remember the diet history is only intended as a snapshot of food intake. It should take not more than 15–20 minutes to record.

(8) Noting family eating habits and preferences is a useful part of the

exercise, giving insight into potential or existing food problem areas.

Having obtained the diet history, count up the number of items chosen from each of the food groups and compare it with the ideal.

Case study
Andrew is a $2\frac{1}{2}$ year old, following the 75th centile for weight and height. Does Andrew's typical food intake for a day, shown in Table 13.1, suggest he is likely to receive an adequate intake of all nutrients?

Table 13.1   Andrew's typical food intake.

Breakfast	$\frac{1}{2}$ slice toast (white), margarine, jam, milky coffee, sugar.
Mid-morning	Chocolate biscuit, diluting juice.
Lunch	Sausage roll, tea biscuits, satsuma, diluting juice.
Mid-afternoon	Packet of chocolate buttons.
Evening	Two fish fingers, chips, $\frac{1}{2}$ yoghurt, tea, sugar.
Bed time	Hot chocolate, made with milk.

Andrew's diet has an appropriate number of servings from milk and dairy foods, therefore his calcium intake is likely to be adequate; intake from the meat, fish and alternatives group is also adequate so protein intake is satisfactory. Although he is not eating enough foods from the bread, other cereals and potatoes group, energy intake is also likely to be satisfactory due to a high consumption of fatty and sugary foods. However, there are likely to be insufficient micronutrients, e.g. iron, since sausage roll and fish fingers are poor sources, and vitamin C since fruit and vegetable intake is low.

In general:

- Lack of variety from any food group and too few choices result in a low intake of major nutrients.
- Too many choices from a food group may result in a poorly balanced diet, i.e. a high intake of some nutrients but a low intake of others.
- Excessive intake of fatty and sugary foods suggests that a diet will provide adequate energy but will be deficient in other nutrients such as vitamins and minerals.

Table 13.2 Andrew's food intake compared with the recommended servings (DoH, 1994) (See Section 12.4 – Meeting nutrient needs).

Food group	Andrew's actual servings	Minimum servings recommended
Milk and dairy foods	$2\frac{1}{2}$	2
Meat, fish and alternatives	2	2 small
Fruit and vegetables	1 fruit No vegetables	1–2 1–2
Bread, other cereals and potatoes	1	4
Fatty and sugary foods	Tea, biscuits, chocolate biscuit, diluting juice, chocolate buttons	Moderate amount of butter, margarine only

Assessing dietary adequacy using the food groups enables advice to be specifically targeted at identified dietary inadequacies.

13.4 Individual nutrients

Accurate analysis of total or single nutrient intake requires assessment by a dietitian, but an estimate of potential dietary adequacy can be made for:

- Calcium
- Iron

13.4.1 Calcium

Toddlers risk an inadequate intake of calcium whenever their intake of milk and milk products is poor. The food groups model indicates that two significant servings (or three or four smaller servings) of milk and dairy foods per day are required where:

1 serving = 180 ml ($\frac{1}{3}$ pint) milk
150 g (5 oz) carton of yoghurt
35 g ($1\frac{1}{4}$ oz) cheddar-type cheese

These are large servings and if three or four smaller servings are taken, calcium needs will be met equally well. A toddler who regularly has fewer than two large or three to four small servings of milk based foods per day risks an inadequate intake.

What can I suggest for a toddler who won't take milk?

- Serve in 'fun' cups or tumblers or encourage the toddler to pour the milk him/herself
- Give milk in 'disguised' but interesting forms, e.g. in sauces, desserts, milk pudding or as a flavoured drink
- Give cheese instead: try the different tastes of Wensleydale, Cheshire, Edam etc. grated or thinly sliced
- Try yoghurts or yoghurt drinks
- Give plenty of other calcium-rich foods such as those in Table 13.3

Advice should be sought from a dietitian if intake of milk and milk products continues to be poor. Calcium supplements may be required.

Table 13.3 Calcium-rich foods.

White bread
Dried fruit (highly cariogenic, see Chapter 10 – Dental Health) e.g. apricots, raisins. Also fruit bread, fruit scones, Garibaldi biscuits.
Fresh or frozen dark green vegetables (spring greens, kale, spinach, green beans, peas, broccoli); try these in soups.
Baked beans.
Other pulses, e.g. lentils (added to cooked rice), butter beans; try in soups.
Peanut butter (smooth variety).
Fromage frais.
Ice cream (sparingly)

13.4.2 Iron

A number of recent studies have shown toddlers to have poor iron status and to be at risk of iron deficiency (Erhardt, 1986; Duggan *et al.*, 1991). This is a cause for concern because iron deficiency, even without overt anaemia, is considered to have an adverse effect on psychomotor development and may also be associated with poor weight gain and increased vulnerability to infection.

Why may iron intake be poor?
Toddlers often have difficulty in achieving an adequate iron intake because:

- Appetite is small
- Iron requirements are high in relation to body size
- Foods which are good sources of readily absorbed iron such as fish, chicken, liver and beef may be eaten infrequently and in small amounts
- With the exception of cereals, iron-fortified infant foods, which provide an iron 'safety net' during the first year, are no longer part of the diet
- Parents are uncertain of suitable iron-rich foods and the variable absorption of iron from different foods
- Parents are unaware of how iron absorption may be enhanced or inhibited by other dietary factors

Table 13.4 Assessing risk factors for a poor iron intake.

Risk factors	Comment
Milk intake in excess of 600 ml (1 pint) per day.	Cow's milk is a poor source of iron and inhibits iron absorption. A high intake reduces appetite for other foods.
Child described as a poor or faddy eater.	Poor total food intake →poor iron intake.
Infrequent consumption of some kind of meat, e.g. < four times per week.	The haem iron of meat is well absorbed, and promotes absorption of iron from other foods.
Iron-fortified breakfast cereal not eaten daily.	Fortified cereals are a valuable source of non-haem iron for toddlers. Encourage consumption with fruit juice or fruit (see below).
Fewer than two servings of fruit or vegetables per day.	Vitimin C promotes iron absorption.
An excessive fibre intake from cereals.	Fibre and phytate in cereals inhibit iron absorption.

Table 13.5 Scoring system for iron assessment.

Food group	Food	Serving	Score
Meat, fish and alternatives (Iron well absorbed)	Liver	2 tbls	8
	Beef mince, casserole	2 tbls	3
	Sliced meat, corned beef	1 slice	1.5
	Beefburger, commercial	1	2
	Lamb, minced, chopped	2 tbls	1.5
	Pork, ham	1 slice	1
	Sausage, bacon	2 small	1
	Meat/fish paste	spread on slice of bread	0.5
	Chicken/turkey	2 tbls	0.5
	Tinned fish, e.g. sardines	2 sardines	4
	Fish finger/other fish	1 finger	1
	Egg	1 small	2
	Baked beans	3 tbls	2
	Lentils	2 tbls	2
	Tahini paste	1.5 tbls	5
	Cooked beans/pulses	2 tbls	2
	Peanut butter	Spread on slice of bread	1
Bread, other cereals and potatoes (Iron less well absorbed)	Iron-fortified breakfast cereal:		
	Weetabix	1 biscuit	2.5
	Cornflakes, Rice Krispies	Child's portion	0.25–2.5
	Ready Brek	Child's portion	2.5
	Bread, wholemeal	1 medium slice	1.5
	white	1 medium slice	0.5
	Pitta bread	1 pitta	2.0
	Chappati	1 med	1.0
	Malt or fruit loaf	1 slice	2.0
	Pasta (boiled)	3 oz	2.5
Fruit and vegetables	Green vegetables	2 tbls	1
	Other vegetables	3 tbls	0.5
	Potato (boiled, baked, chips)	1 egg sized or 7 chips	0.5
	Dried fruit	3 tbls	1.5
Milk and dairy foods	Milk*		
	Infant formulae	1 beaker	3
	Follow-on formulae	1 beaker	6
	Fruit yoghurt	1 carton	1

Continued

Table 13.5 Continued

Food group	Food	Serving	Score
Fatty/sugary foods (Not a recommended source of iron, but should be taken into account)	Chocolate biscuit	1 biscuit	2
	Chocolate	1 small bar	2
	Crisps	small pkt.	1.5
	Sponge cake/pudding	1 small slice	1
	Plain sweet biscuit	1 biscuit	0.5
	Liquorice	2 shoelaces	1.5

*Cow's milk and milk products have a negligible iron content. 'Toddler' milk drinks may be fortified with iron, e.g. follow-on milks.

Table 13.6 Using the scoring system in Table 13.5.

Infant (7–12 months) score	Toddler (1–3 years) score	Recommendation
> 26	> 23	Diet contains adequate iron
20–26	18–23	Average iron requirements are likely to be met, but children with high requirements risk deficiency
< 20	< 18	Iron intake likely to be unsatisfactory: • Encourage greater intake of iron-rich foods • Consider referral for dietetic assessment
< 14	< 12	Iron intake unsatisfactory: • Refer for dietary assessment

From: Southern Derbyshire Health Authority, 1993. (Adapted from Table 6 with permission from Dr L. Hyde.)

Assessing iron adequacy

The following provides a means of assessing the potential iron adequacy of a toddler's diet:

(1) Risk factors:

• Assess the toddler's diet in respect of the risk factors for a poor iron intake (Table 13.4).

(2)   Assess iron intake
- 'Score' the toddler's diet according to his iron intake
- Record a single day diet history (see Section 13.3.1)
- Calculate the iron score of the diet using Table 13.5
- Take appropriate action

All portions in Table 13.5 have been estimated as toddler-sized, small, or single items, e.g. 1 cracker, 1 slice of bread, 1 slice of meat.

14. Eating for Future Health

'In a nutshell, the problem is how to change the diet of an unweaned baby from a fibre free, high fat intake to a high fibre, low fat diet by 5.'

Taitz, 1987

This chapter covers:

- The rationale for encouraging healthy eating early
- The extent to which adult dietary targets can be applied to young children
- Practical advice on reducing fat, sugar and salt intake
- Practical advice on an appropriate intake of fibre rich foods

There is a lack of comprehensive dietary recommendations for young children aged 1–5 years. Current dietary recommendations for **adults** are to eat more:

- Vegetables
- Fruit
- Bread
- Breakfast cereals
- Potatoes
- Rice
- Pasta

and to aim for variety in our food.

Such changes are seen as the means of reducing the incidence of diet-related diseases and mortality in the adult population, and dietary recommendations are specified in the COMA report on dietary reference values (DoH, 1991).

The targets in Table 14.1 cannot be applied strictly to young children because of the risk of compromising nutrient intake, but healthy eating habits should be encouraged from an early age.

Why encourage healthy eating so early?

Many risk factors for coronary heart disease (CHD) – obesity,

Table 14.1 Targets for the adult population.

	% of total energy/day
Total fat intake of which saturated fat Starches, intrinsic sugars and milk sugars Non-milk extrinsic sugars	< 35 < 11 > 40 < 10
Non-starch polysaccharide (fibre)	> 16g/day
Sodium	70 mmols/day

From: The Scottish Diet, Table 5.2. Scottish Office, 1993.

hypertension and hypercholesterolaemia – have their origins in child-hood (Taitz & Wardley, 1990; Deckelbaum, 1990) (see Appendix I). Parental control over a child's food intake is greatest in the first few years of life and at this age parents can favourably influence food preferences. Good habits established early can exert a long-term positive influence on food choice.

Dietary modifications of fat and fibre need not have a detrimental effect on the growth of pre-school children (Payne & Belton, 1992a). However, parents require practical suggestions for the appropriate application of adult healthy eating guidelines.

14.1 Fat

Diets with a high percentage of energy from saturated fat are associated with an increased risk of CHD. However, fat is an important source of energy, essential fatty acids and vitamins A and D for young children. Fat is also important for making foods more palatable.

Can I advise a reduction in fat intake?
Nutritious high fat foods should not be limited and Table 14.2 describes appropriate use of these foods. Limit intake of high fat foods such as chips, fried foods, pastry products, crisps, chocolate, sweet biscuits and cakes; these foods are of low nutritional value and a high intake may result in excessive energy intake and weight gain.

14.2 Fibre

Dietary fibre is important for the long-term health of the gut and prevents constipation. Foods containing fibre supply a variety of

Table 14.2 Nutritious high fat foods.

Milk	Provides energy, calcium, protein, vitamins. Give whole milk until two years. Semi-skimmed milk can be given from two years if growth is satisfactory. Skimmed milk should not be given until five years.
Cheese, dairy products	Provides energy, protein, calcium, vitamins. Use regularly in meals and snacks. Do not give low fat varieties before two years.
Meats	Important source of protein, iron, zinc. Choose leaner meats whenever possible. Trim off visible fat. Grill instead of fry. Limit intake of fatty meat products, e.g. sausage roll, pie, sausages. Do not avoid meat without seeking dietary advice.
Oily fish	Oily fish (sardines, pilchards, salmon, kipper, herring etc.) are good sources of protein, unsaturated fat and calcium. Give regularly.
Spreading fats	Spreading fats – provide energy and vitamins. Spread butter and margarine thinly. Choose polyunsaturated margarine to cut down on saturated fat. Do not give low fat spreads before two years Do not cut out spreading fat before five years.
Oils	Provide vitamins, energy. Choose unsaturated oils (sunflower, soya, vegetable, olive, rapeseed) in preference to hard fats. Limit fried food.
Nuts	Do *not* give whole nuts to children under five years (due to risk of choking). Smooth peanut butter and tahini are good sources of energy and calcium.

vitamins and minerals. However, a high fibre diet can be bulky and of low nutrient density. Excessive fibre intakes can also interfere with absorption of minerals and can sometimes cause diarrhoea or intestinal discomfort.

What can I advise about fibre?

Provided a child is growing well and is consuming a satisfactory number of servings from each of the following – milk and dairy foods; meat, fish and alternatives; bread, other cereals and potatoes – then he or she may gradually be introduced to high fibre foods. Table 14.3 gives guidance on the gradual introduction of fibre containing foods. Avoid very large quantities of fruit and vegetables or raw, unprocessed bran.

Table 14.3 Fibre in a toddler's diet.

Cereals	Give wholemeal or grain breads instead of white or brown. Encourage fibre-rich breakfast cereals (e.g. Raisin Wheats, Mini-Shreddies, Weetabix). Try whole-wheat pasta. Give oatcakes and wholegrain crackers as snacks.
Vegetables	Give 1–2 portions daily. Choose fresh, frozen or tinned. Include in soups and casseroles.
Fruits	Give 1–2 portions daily. Leave skins on whenever appropriate. Give dried fruit (contains iron) regularly.
Pulses	Use regularly and try different varieties (butter beans, chick peas, lentils) as well as baked beans.

14.3 Sugar

The recommendation to reduce sugar intake refers to non-milk extrinsic (NME) sugars (see Chapter 10 – Dental Health). In practical terms, this means all sugars other than those found in fruit and milk. (Fruit juice contains NMEs.) Sugar is unnecessary as a source of energy in the diet because all starchy foods are digested to supply glucose, the body's main energy source. Sugar supplies no nutrients other than calories, and frequent consumption of foods containing sugar is associated with a high risk of dental caries because the neutralising capacity of saliva is inhibited. (For the process of dental decay see Chapter 10).

Sugars + mouth bacteria → acid → demineralisation = risk of decay
Frequent NME sugars + mouth bacteria → frequent acid →
prolonged demineralisation = high risk of decay

What can I advise about sugar?

Much of the advice on sugars and dental health in Chapter 10 is applicable to toddlers and pre-school children. The following suggestions incorporating this advice can be made:

(1) Limit the **frequency** with which sweet foods and drinks are given and do not allow them to be consumed over a prolonged period.
(2) Do not manipulate toddlers by using sweet foods as bribes, rewards or consolation.
(3) Replace high sugar foods with lower sugar alternatives; suggestions for achieving this are given in Table 14.4. Other ideas can be found in Chapter 21 – Feeding Problems.
(4) Avoid reinforcing a preference for sweet foods through excessive use of artificially sweetened foods and drinks such as fizzy drinks, yoghurts and dessert mixes. High intake of artificial sweeteners, derived from such foods, is not recommended for young children (see Chapter 24 – Additives).
(5) Establish good dental habits to include twice daily tooth brushing and regular dental check-ups.
(6) Be aware of different names for sugar. These are listed in Section 10.4.4.

When can sugary foods be eaten?

If due attention is paid to dental health, some sugar in foods at meal times is perfectly acceptable and provides a toddler with useful amounts of energy. Foods such as cornflakes, fruit scone, tomato soup, baked beans and rice pudding contain sugar but supply other important nutrients and should not be discouraged.

14.4 Salt

Sodium in food is mainly in the form of salt. A high salt intake is associated with an increase in blood pressure with increasing age in susceptible individuals. Children's blood pressures already display the tendency to rise with age (Rose *et al.*, 1989). There is very little risk of healthy toddlers in Britain becoming sodium depleted following a moderation in family salt intake, and therefore this is recommended.

Table 14.4 Sweet food alternatives.

High sugar foods	Lower sugar alternative foods
Chocolate, sugar or honey coated breakfast cereals	Rice Krispies, Cornflakes or Raisin Wheats with fruit e.g. banana, raisins
Jam, honey, chocolate spread, lemon curd	Reduced sugar jam, Marmite (sparingly), peanut butter, cheese spread
Juice drinks and squashes, fizzy drinks	Water, fresh fruit juice diluted with water, sugar-free squash.
Chocolate and very sweet biscuits	Plainer biscuits, e.g. rich tea, crackers, oatcakes, bread sticks, cheesy biscuits
Sticky cakes and pastries	Scones, fruit bread, rock buns, banana loaf (low sugar varieties)
Tinned fruit in syrup	Tinned fruit in juice, fresh fruit
Milk shakes, bought yoghurt drinks	Milk + fresh fruit, e.g. banana; milk + yoghurt
Chewy sweets, toffees, candies	Small quantity of dried fruit*, e.g. raisins, apple rings, apricots; fruit bar; chocolate**.

* Dried fruit is more cariogenic than fresh fruit (fruit sugar is concentrated by drying and dried fruit is 'sticky' to teeth). However, it is less cariogenic than sweets and provides minerals.
** Chocolate is potentially less cariogenic than chewy type sweets, but still contains a lot of sugar.

What can I advise about salt?

Limit salty snacks such as crisps, corn or wheat snacks, cheesy puffs, salted popcorn.

Whole nuts should not be given under 5 years.

See Chapter 23 – Meals and Snacks, for snack ideas.

Avoid unnecessary use of salt in cooking and food preparation. Use only small quantities in cooking and avoid adding salt to food at table routinely.

Most dietary salt (i.e. 85%) is obtained from bought foods, two thirds of which is added during manufacturing (James *et al.*, 1987). Therefore limit the use of processed foods; whenever possible use fresh fruit, fresh or frozen vegetables, pasta and rice. Choose lower salt varieties of processed foods when available, e.g. vegetables tinned without salt. Use flavourings such as stock cubes, gravy granules and Marmite sparingly. These all have a high salt content. Avoid the use of salt substitutes such as Lo-salt.

Do not be over-concerned about giving some salt-containing processed foods. Many foods, e.g. baked beans, tinned fish, spaghetti shapes, cheese spread, are a valuable source of nutrients in a toddler's diet.

14.5 Summary

Adult healthy eating guidelines are not directly applicable to toddlers and should not be rigidly applied to their diets. There is no such thing as the ideal healthy diet. Decisions have to be made regarding fat, fibre, sugar and salt intakes which will not compromise dietary adequacy. Occasional consumption of high fat/high sugar/high salt foods does not make a diet unhealthy, but daily or frequent consumption of such foods can set an unwelcome pattern for later life.

Efforts to achieve dietary goals will inevitably be modified by social, economic and cultural pressures. Individually targeted advice is always required. Example is important: toddlers have to learn dietary habits – both good and bad.

15. Meal Time Considerations

> 'Food should be enjoyable and eating and drinking can, and should, be socially valuable.'
>
> Walker & Cannon, 1984

This chapter covers:

- A toddler's perspective of meal times
- The importance of a calm meal time environment.

Toddlers are renowned for being 'faddy' or 'problem' eaters but meal time battles can often be prevented by consideration of the toddlers' perspective of meal times and appropriate forward planning.

15.1 Feeding development

For toddlers, eating is as much a learning as a refuelling process. Meal times allow for the development of eating skills and improved dexterity, the development of socially acceptable behaviour and the experience of different food tastes and combinations. Eating skills, however, take time to develop and practise. Table 15.1 illustrates this.

What about...?

The mess?
Inevitable, but damage limitation is straightforward: bib, rolled-up sleeves, sheet on the floor etc.

Finger-feeding?
Should not be discouraged too quickly. Finger foods allow easy self-feeding and can encourage increased interest in eating.

Eating at a table?
Table eating with other family members is to be strongly encouraged; this provides routine and promotes learning by example and use of cutlery.

Table 15.1 Development of eating skills.

Age	Skills
1 year	Uses a drinking cup with help. Holds a spoon, but not able to load it or reach mouth without spillage. Predominantly finger feeding. Messy. Needs high chair/booster cushion at table.
18 months	Manages a cup unaided. Holds a spoon securely, reasonably reliable in feeding. Messy. Needs high chair/alternative.
2 years	Chews food well. Spoon feeds well. Sucks (not chews!) from a straw. Tidier. Needs high chair/alternative.
3 years	Cuts soft food with a knife. Uses fingers, spoon, fork, cup. Self feeding with assistance, e.g. to cut meat. Generally tidy. Sits at table, but tendency to get down and run around..
4+	Competent use of knife and fork.

Positioning?
Positioning of a toddler in relation to the table and his food must enable him to get at the food easily.

Example?
Because much of learning is by example, parents and other family members are important meal time role models.

Independence?
Important to toddlers. A balance needs to be struck between helping to feed and self-feeding. Too much assisted feeding may result in a 'lazy' eater.

Nutrition?
Toddlers commonly spend a lot of time and energy at meal times but

may not eat very much (repeatedly loading food on to a spoon and losing the contents, playing with cutlery, lifting a drinking cup). This is not a cause for concern. Toddler energy requirements decline with increasing age, and total nutrient intake per day is generally larger than parents imagine.

15.2 Meal time environment

The meal time environment needs to encourage eating. Disturbed and noisy meal times or background distractions are not helpful. An ideal eating environment would include:

- Eating at a table with the rest of the family, not in front of television or 'on the move'
- Routines to build familiarity
- Appropriate toddler utensils
- No background distractions
- An unhurried approach
- Removal of uneaten food without fuss

15.3 Food appeal

Food presentation is as important for young children as it is to adults eating in a restaurant. Colour, shape, garnish and contrast all serve to make food look attractive and therefore worthy of further investigation. Toddler meals need to be kept as simple as possible to save parental frustration, but there are many simple ways of increasing meal appeal.

Portions
Large portions can be very off-putting and may result in refusal to eat any of the meal. Portions should be small and different foods separated on a plate so that they can be seen and recognised.

Colour
Colour and colour contrast are vital. Foods which are brown, beige, off-white and sludge green have little visual appeal served singly or together, whereas foods which are red, green, orange or yellow provide lively contrasts. Table 15.2 gives examples of suitable colourful foods which also tend to contain useful vitamins. Table 15.3 compares the colour contrasts of different meals.

Table 15.2 Colourful foods.

Reds	Greens	Oranges	Yellows
Tomato, tomato purée, radish, kidney beans, peppers, strawberries, red-skinned apple.	Broccoli, cabbage, peas, green beans etc. cress, cucumber, parsley, kiwi fruit, apple.	Carrots, cooked swede, baked beans, spaghetti shapes, fish fingers, cheese, satsuma, tinned peaches.	Cheese slices, egg yolk, sweetcorn, pineapple.

Table 15.3 Colour contrasts of different meals.

Meal	Colours
Bacon and corn pizza with cucumber slices	Pink, yellow, red, green
Mince with cauliflower and potato	Brown and white
Fish finger with peas and potato	Orange, green, white
Sausage roll and chips	Brown/beige

Shape and size

Different shapes and sizes of food make it more interesting and some shapes lend themselves to easy eating with fingers. Examples are given in Table 15.4. Many purchased foods are also available with shape appeal, e.g. tinned or dried pasta shapes, alphabet oven chips, potato waffles.

Some parents may even consider using foods to make more complicated shape pictures. This is time-consuming but can encourage eating (see Table 15.5). Similar ideas are to be found in parentcraft magazines and cookery books. A number of such books are listed in the Recommended Reading section at the back of the book.

15.4 Eating location

There is a lot to be said in favour of changing the eating location occasionally, which can add interest to meal times and make eating an

Table 15.4   Finger foods.

Shape	Examples
Sticks/fingers	Cut vegetables, e.g. carrots, cucumber, courgette, celery. Fruit, e.g. apple, pear. Toast fingers, breadsticks, sponge finger, tea biscuit, cheese, low fat chips.
Wedges	Cheese, cheese triangles, tomato, cucumber.
'Mini foods'	Cherry tomatoes, new potatoes, seedless grapes. Mini varieties of cheesy biscuits, oatcakes, rice cakes, Shreddies, pizzas, crumpets or pancakes; boxes of raisins; chipolatas, burger bites, mini sandwiches.

activity, social event or adventure. Children who tend to be reluctant eaters often eat well when away from the usual meal time location, e.g. on holiday, with grandparents. Even good eaters benefit from variety, and alternative locations include:

- In the garden or park
- In a make-shift 'café' at home
- With other toddlers at playschool
- At a friend's or relative's house

Table 15.5   Food pictures.

Picture	Examples
Cutouts	Use of biscuit cutters to make mini sandwiches or pizza shapes, French toast animals, toast/biscuit people.
Fish	Fish-shaped fish-cakes, fish-shaped filled puff pastry cases.
Boats	$\frac{1}{2}$ baked potato/crumpet/roll with filling or topping and a 'sail'.
Faces (preferably smiling!)	On pizza, potato-topped pie, using vegetables for nose, eyes and mouth, or drawn on to a boiled egg shell.

15.5 Food as an activity

Allowing children to play with and handle food from an early age is a recognised way of promoting interest in food. Encourage parents to let toddlers become involved in safe food play. This becomes more relevant in older pre-school children (3–5 years).

Food play suggestions

- Playing with a variety of coloured and textured foods
- 'Washing' vegetables
- Cutting out pastry shapes with plastic cutters
- 'Pretend' tea parties
- Using empty food cartons as building blocks

16. Feeding Problems

> 'No child has ever starved to death through stubbornness.'
>
> Green, 1992

This chapter covers:

- The psychological nature of food refusal
- Factors associated with refusal to eat
- Advice on how to reduce parents' anxiety about food refusal

Feeding problems are remarkably common among young children. An estimated 12–34% of toddlers and pre-school children are believed to be 'difficult eaters' (Minde & Minde, 1986).

Two broad types of feeding problems exist:

(1)   Refusal to eat
(2)   Excessive faddiness

Food refusal is considered first, along with a number of other food behaviour problems. Excessive faddiness is considered in Chapter 21.

16.1   Food refusal

What causes toddler food refusal?
A small minority of children may have either minor organic disorders or underlying disease states which could result in feeding difficulties or food aversion which give rise to food refusal. Such conditions include oral motor dysfunction, cerebral palsy, cancer and/or chemotherapy treatment.

In the majority of cases there is no organic cause for toddler food refusal and the reasons for refusal to eat are psychologically based.

Medical conditions must always be considered and excluded as a reason for a child failing to eat.

In the absence of underlying disease or disorder, toddlers may refuse to eat for the following reasons:

- Poor appetite
- Limited food appeal
- Emotional upset
- Manipulative behaviour

Appetite

Toddlers require less energy per kg body weight than infants, and older toddlers require less energy than younger toddlers. Appetite decreases correspondingly. Small energy intakes are perfectly compatible with normal growth. In addition, individual appetite and energy requirements differ greatly. A 1992 study of pre-school children found 100% difference in maximum energy intakes in two and three year olds (Payne & Belton, 1992a).

A toddler may not be hungry due to:

- Small appetite
- Excessive intake of snacks or drinks, especially milk
- Feeling unwell
- Constipation
- An 'off' day: toddler appetites are not constant
- Anxiety or upset

Limited food appeal

Food may be found to be unappealing for a number of reasons:

- *Looks or smells different* – young children show a strong preference for familiar rather than novel foods. This 'fear' of new tastes is a normal part of development (Skuse, 1993).
- *Looks difficult to chew* – poor chewing skills are common in children not introduced to foods containing 'lumps' during weaning before 6–7 months.
- *Too much on the plate* – this is a strong disincentive to adult eating, and its significance needs to be recognised.
- *Looks unappealing* – colour and contrast provide important visual incentive to eat (see Section 15.3).
- *Genuinely disliked* – toddlers have well established taste preferences and, similar to adults, established likes and dislikes. These should be respected.

Emotional upset

Toddler behaviour is strongly influenced by past experience. Any negative experience of food or meal times will result in behaviour directed at avoiding a similar experience. Such experiences might include an episode of choking, an adverse reaction to a food or force feeding. Toddlers, like adults, can also use food, or rejection of food, as an emotional outlet to express anxiety or seek attention following an upset. This could be a major life disruption such as the birth of a sibling, or something relatively trivial.

Manipulative development

Food refusal is considered by some experts to be a normal expression of the need for independence (Francis, 1986). Toddler meal times are as much a learning experience as a time for eating; the determination to self-feed allows development of feeding skills.

Refusing food can equally be a useful means for a toddler to get what he or she wants, such as increased attention or a preferred food item. Manipulative food refusal is common and often follows food refusal for other reasons. If a favourable outcome is achieved as a result of food refusal, then the behaviour is positively reinforced, i.e. it is made worthwhile repeating. Thus the parents' response to food refusal often serves to exacerbate the problem (Fig. 16.1).

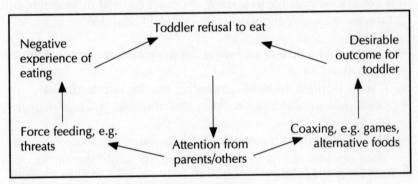

Fig. 16.1 Reinforcement of food refusal.

16.1.1 Management of food refusal

Management involves:

(1) Excluding organic cause of refusal to eat
(2) Consideration of non-organic causes
(3) Reducing parental anxiety
(4) Refusing to do battle on toddler terms

(1) Excluding organic cause of food refusal
Weight and height measurements should always be made for any child presenting with food refusal.

- Plot weight and height in child health record
- Ask about: child's general wellbeing:
  - bowel habits
  - sleep pattern
  - history of recent illness
  - past medical conditions
- If the child's growth is poor and/or symptoms are described, referral should be made to a paediatrician
- If growth is adequate and the child is symptom-free, organic cause is unlikely

Prolonged food refusal, due to non-organic causes can result in impaired growth. Regular weight monitoring should be carried out to ensure growth adequacy. Vitamin drops should be given in all cases of food refusal.

(2) Consideration of non-organic causes
It is not always possible to identify the exact cause(s) of food refusal, but discussion with parent(s) or carers should consider:

- Family eating habits including food preferences, meal pattern, location of eating
- Toddlers daily food intake: including snacks, sweets, drinks
- Onset and duration of feeding problems, and potential 'trigger' events
- Parents and others response to food refusal.

Sometimes easily remedied causes can be found such as with a toddler too full with milk/sweets/snacks to eat his meal, but often cases are more complex.

(3) Reducing parental anxiety
Reducing anxiety is the key to resolving the majority of toddler food refusal problems. Parents are understandably anxious and frustrated when a child refuses to eat and, for the majority of parents, their main concern is for the child's health. In the parents' minds prolonged food refusal will lead to illness and malnutrition and possibly the death of the child.

This major underlying concern may then be exacerbated by frustration at the time taken to prepare food and the cost of wasted meals; plus frustration at the child's bad behaviour, and anxiety about 'failing' as a parent, or appearing to neglect the child. Anxiety therefore tends to govern parents' response to food refusal behaviour.

To reduce parental anxiety:

- Plot height and weight on the child's record chart to reassure in respect of growth and adequacy (refer child for medical assessment if required).
- Explore current dietary intake and highlight positive aspects.
- Explain that toddler requirements are less than infant requirements.
- Reassure that the child is extremely unlikely to starve himself to death and that a diet which is temporarily bizarre will do no harm.
- Recommend vitamin drops are given.
- Emphasise that food refusal *always* resolves eventually, but it may take time to do so.
- For parents who are excessively concerned, or where the long term nutritional adequacy of the diet is in question, arrange for the child to be referred to a dietitian. Even minor dietary modifications can help to alleviate parental anxiety if food intake is perceived to be increased.

The underlying goal of managing food refusal should be to remove the stress associated with meal times. Reducing parents' anxiety goes a long way towards this. The discussion in Chapter 15 – Meal Time Considerations – is also relevant.

(4) Refusing to do battle on toddler terms
Parents need to understand the importance of not responding to toddler food behaviour. The best policy, although extremely hard to implement, is to *ignore* it.

The following ten point plan of action is recommended:

(1) Give regular meals seated at a table with the television switched off.
(2) Prepare simple meals (to minimise frustration if rejected).
(3) To start with, give foods known to be well-accepted.
(4) Give small quantities, presented separately.
(5) Ignore food refusal:
   - **Do not** coax to eat

- **Do not** force to eat
- **Do not** get upset

(6) When it is obvious no more food is going to be eaten, remove it and allow the child to leave the table.

(7) Do not offer preferred alternatives or sweet foods.

(8) Ignore all bad behaviour.

(9) Praise highly if food is eaten and get other family members to do likewise.

(10) Allow toddler to eat with other 'good eater' toddlers whenever possible.

16.2   Other food-related problems

16.2.1   Vomiting on demand

Vomiting on demand must be distinguished from vomiting due to underlying disease. This requires attention to the vomiting history and the wellbeing of the child.

Vomiting on demand is a talent that comes easily to many young children. It is an effective means of parent manipulation because it is so dramatic. Vomiting may be associated with rejection of certain foods, but may equally be used to manipulate on other issues such as bed-times. Vomiting is often arrived at by way of prolonged crying. Vomiting behaviour may be learned in infancy either as a result of reflux vomiting or, occasionally, as part of a poor parent–child bonding syndrome (Harris & Booth, 1992).

Vomiting on demand is rarely a cause of nutritional concern, but may require consideration of social and emotional family issues.

What should I advise?
Where vomiting on demand is evidently manipulative, the following advice is appropriate:

- Do not manipulate the diet in an effort to prevent vomiting.
- Abandon all efforts to force-feed or coax eating and follow strategy for food refusal.
- Allow persistent criers to cry for a short time before offering a small amount of comfort, but not excessive attention. Repeat this strategy if necessary.
- Clean the child who has vomited without anger, emotion or any 'quality' attention.

- Due attention must be given to safety and cleanliness, but habitual vomiting, like food refusal, improves only through ignoring it.

16.2.2   Refusing to chew

There is a well recognised 'sensitive' period for the introduction of solid food. Failure to introduce texture and lumps before 6–7 months of age commonly results in the rejection of lumpy food later on (Illingworth & Lister, 1964). Prolonged use of untextured (Stage I type) baby foods is a common cause of 'lump aversion' and lack of experience of chewing may cause gagging when it is attempted, reinforcing the inclination not to chew.

Refusal to chew may be due, in part, to stubbornness relating to a preference for the taste of manufactured foods, or a disinclination to pursue chewing skills. Unsurprisingly, biscuits, chocolate or toast are often chewed readily!

What should I advise?

- Do not allow milk intake to exceed 1 pint per day (often used as a substitute food).
- Start by adding some home-prepared liquidised food to favourite tinned baby foods.
- Gradually make food more home-made, including soft lumps.
- Encourage finger foods, which are often more acceptable.
- Avoid serving lumps which cannot be recognised.

16.2.3   Refusing to give up breast or bottle

Refusal to stop breast or bottle feeding may be an indication that a toddler has come to see the breast or bottle as an object or habit of comfort. Use of breast or bottle feeds as a comforter should be discouraged because a feed may become a prerequisite for sleep, and night feeding is associated with night waking (and wet nappies). Prolonged bottle or breastfeeding (beyond 18 months) is associated with an increased risk of tooth decay. Similarly, feeding from a bottle beyond one year encourages the 'wandering around' habit, whereby milk or juice drinks can be prolonged over several hours. This is associated with a high risk of tooth decay.

What should I advise?

- Try to identify the pattern of continuous breast or bottle feeding. Is it, for example, for all drinks, at night or only when tired or upset?
- Restrict feeds initially to one or two specific times per day.
- Give a feeding cup (with a lid if required) at all other times.
- Give plenty of attention.
- Substitute other comforters, e.g. soft toy or blanket when comfort and not drink is needed.
- Do not give in to tantrums; stick to a strategy.
- Be patient; weaning a toddler may take time.

17.   Other Common Concerns

> 'Certain nutritionally related problems which occur in otherwise normal children are not manifestations of serious illness, but are a serious cause of inconvenience and potential anxiety.'
>
> Taitz and Wardley, 1990

This chapter covers:

- Practical advice on the management of toddler diarrhoea
- Practical advice on the management of constipation
- Government recommendations on the use of supplementary welfare vitamins

17.1   Toddler diarrhoea

Toddler diarrhoea without failure to thrive (chronic, non-specific diarrhoea) is the most common form of diarrhoea in childhood (Walker-Smith, 1980). Toddler diarrhoea is characterised by:

- Onset between 6 and 24 months of age, resolving with time between 2 and 4 years
- Frequent loose and watery stools, often containing particles of undigested food
- Continued weight gain and wellbeing of the child

What causes diarrhoea?

The exact cause of toddler diarrhoea is not known but disordered intestinal motility is found to exist in many cases and this is believed to be of relevance in the pathogenesis of the disorder. A high incidence of bowel dysfunction has also been noted in the parents of affected children (Davidson & Wasserman, 1966). Other contributory factors may be the reduction in fat intake which occurs at weaning, causing faster gastric emptying, and minor recurrent infections. A high fruit and/or fruit juice intake can cause osmotic diarrhoea. Excessive squash drinking is also implicated as a cause of loose stools (Green & Gishan, 1983).

There is little evidence to suggest that toddler diarrhoea is due to food sensitivity and this is not a theory supported by current expert opinion (Walker-Smith, 1987).

Management
Management centres on reassuring parents that toddler diarrhoea is transitory. Extensive medical investigations and drug therapy are not appropriate. Since many children referred with toddler diarrhoea do have a low dietary fat intake, increasing the fat intake can be beneficial. Regulating the fluid intake of excessive drinkers has also been found to be helpful.

Practical action
- Measure weight, length and head circumference to assess growth adequacy, and if growth is poor, or the child is unwell, refer for medical assessment.
- If growth is adequate and the child appears well, refer for stool culture and check for reducing substances (indicative of lactose intolerance).
- Reassure parents that the diarrhoea, although distressing, is not a cause for concern.
- Emphasise that it is a transitory condition and will resolve in time (usually *before* the start of nursery school).
- Assess approximate fat intake. Where appropriate recommend increasing dietary fat intake to include 1 pint of *whole* milk per day, and increased use of spreading fat, cheese and higher fat foods.
- Assess approximate fruit and fibre intake. Where appropriate recommend reducing intake of wholegrain cereal foods, reducing intake of fruit juice and limiting fruit intake to one serving per day.
- Warn parents against embarking on dietary restriction in an effort to control diarrhoea since this can compromise nutritional intake.
- Refer to a dietitian for full dietary assessment if required.

17.2   Constipation
Bowel problems in children are common and problems with constipation often occur when toilet training is in progress. Chronic constipation may be associated with soiling, which can be particularly distressing for both parents and the toddler. The cause of constipation is usually multifactorial. Reluctance to evacuate the bowel may be due to:

- Distress or pain associated with previous efforts
- Fear of the potty or toilet
- Being too busy to respond to the appropriate signals

Constipation may also be due in part to a child having a naturally sluggish bowel.

Parental anxiety about toilet training and the commonly found obsession with bowel habits can act to exacerbate the situation and it is important to remind parents that toddlers, like adults, show great natural variety in their bowel habits.

Management
Management of constipation depends on its severity, i.e. duration and the child's previous history. Dietary advice is relevant in the majority of cases. Many constipated children are found to be poor eaters and to drink up to 2 litres of milk per day (Clayden, 1992).

What can I advise?
For an isolated episode of milk constipation, i.e. 2–3 days duration if daily bowel habit is the norm, suggest:

- Drinks of pure fruit juice two to three times per day (prune juice is particularly effective)
- Giving a high fibre breakfast cereal, e.g. Weetabix, Branflakes, mixed in with regular cereal
- Increasing fluid intake (other than milk) to at least six cups per day
- Sitting the child on the toilet after each meal

If this fails to work, suggest a mild children's laxative and give advice regarding fibre intake so as to avoid further episodes.

For more severe, chronic constipation laxatives are generally required and since the type and dose depend on the severity of the constipation, medical referral is recommended.

The unsupervised or regular use of laxatives is to be avoided.

Overuse of laxatives will exacerbate the problem of a sluggish bowel by creating dependency on their use. Furthermore, it does not address toilet training problems and can cause loss of important minerals from the body.

17.3   Supplementary government vitamins

Why are they necessary?

Individual vitamins are required in small amounts but an adequate vitamin intake is essential for good health. A toddler eating a varied diet, containing foods from each of the food groups, is likely to have an adequate intake and satisfactory vitamin status. However, toddlers who are faddy or poor eaters will have variable intakes. Vitamin adequacy can be estimated from food intake, but not guaranteed. Government recommendations state:

> 'Between the ages of one and five years, vitamin A and D supplements should be given unless adequate vitamin status can be assured.'

> (DoH, 1994)

In the majority of cases it is very difficult to be certain that vitamin status is satisfactory.

The provision of vitamin D in this way is an important means of protecting against vitamin D deficiency. It is difficult for a toddler to achieve an adequate intake of vitamin D from food, and skin synthesis of the vitamin is unreliable in Britain, especially during winter. Asian infants and young children are at particularly high risk of deficiency and should always be given government (welfare) vitamin drops in the recommended dosage of five drops daily. The provision of welfare vitamins is detailed in Appendix III.

Vitamin supplements should be offered with food, but avoided if the child is not eating.

Are they safe?

There is minimal danger of a toddler exceeding a safe intake of vitamins A, C and D when government drops are given in the recommended dosage. This is true even if dietary intake is good or if follow-on milk (which is supplemented with the same vitamins) is being used. However, there is evidence to suggest that parents are not always clear about either the correct dosage or the potential dangers of overdosage with vitamin drops. Clear guidance must be given regarding the appropriate and safe use of vitamin supplements.

What about other vitamin preparations?

A 1992 study found that 30% of parents who gave their children extra vitamins obtained them from sources other than child health clinics (Ko *et al.*, 1992). This is undesirable because:

- There is increased potential for overdosage
- Parents' awareness of potential toxicity is often poor
- Commercial vitamin preparations may be used as a substitute for dietary improvement

Overdosing is uncommon, but it is not unknown (Evans & Lacey, 1986) and parents should be made aware of the risks of overdosage. Water soluble vitamins, e.g. vitamin C, taken in excess of need are excreted in the urine, but high intakes of fat soluble vitamins are retained and an excess is toxic (see Table 17.1).

Table 17.1 Vitamin overdosage.

Vitamin	Potential outcome of excessive intake
Vitamin A	Hypertension, brain injury
Vitamin D	Hypercalcaemia, renal damage
Vitamin C	Haematina (in huge doses)
Vitamin B_6	Peripheral neuropathy

Do vitamins increase intelligence?
There is no convincing evidence to support this claim. The results of studies which linked high intakes of vitamins to increased IQ have not been substantiated. Similarly, the claim that high intakes of vitamin C protect against the development of colds is unproven. Giving large doses of vitamins for such reasons is not recommended.

Summary
Government vitamin drops are recommended for all children from one year, and preferably up to five years. Parents who choose not to give government vitamin drops should be made aware of the potential risks of vitamin D deficiency, and the need to give a balanced and varied diet. Additional vitamins should *not* be given to toddlers receiving government vitamin drops. This practice risks overdosage. Parents who choose to give commercial vitamin preparations should be made aware of the dangers of overdosage. Only children's products should

be given and the manufacturers' recommended dosage should not be exceeded.

17.4   *Hyperactivity*

Hyperactivity is covered fully in Section 24.3.1

18. Vegetarian and Ethnic Minority Diets

> 'A well-planned vegetarian diet can be nutritionally adequate and health promoting for both adults and children.'
>
> British Dietetic Association, 1995

This chapter covers:

- Nutritional implications of different vegetarian diets
- Reasons why children of ethnic minorities may be at increased risk of nutritional deficiencies.

18.1 Introduction

The UK is now a country of great cultural and ethnic diversity. This has contributed to increasing dietary diversity. Vegetarianism is common among many ethnic groups and is found increasingly in the indigenous population. Vegetarian and ethnic diets are largely compatible with normal child growth, but some practices may compromise dietary adequacy.

The following is an overview of dietary variants found within the UK, and their potential nutritional problems. However, since the specific needs of different groups are affected by local factors and vary greatly, information relating to the dietary habits of ethnic groups should be sought from within individual localities, e.g. community dietetic departments. Sources of further information are given in the Resources List at the back of the book.

18.2 Vegetarian and vegan diets

18.2.1 Definitions and backgrounds

Vegetarianism is practised for a variety of religious, cultural, philosophical and social reasons and involves varying degrees of dietary restriction. The term vegetarian requires clarification with individual families. Definitions are:

- *Lacto-ovo vegetarian* – Excludes all meat, fish, poultry
- *Lacto vegetarian* – Excludes all meat, fish, poultry, eggs
- *Vegan* – Consumes no food of animal origin

The nutritional implications of these variants are given in Table 18.1. The term vegetarian is used in the following text to describe lacto and lacto-ovo vegetarian.

Table 18.1 Classification of vegetarianism and veganism.

	Foods excluded	Protein source		Nutrient at risk of deficiency
Partial vegetarian	Red meat Offal	Poultry Fish Milk Cheese Yoghurt	Eggs Beans Lentils	Iron (Energy)
Lacto-ovo vegetarian	Red meat Offal Fish Poultry	Milk Cheese Yoghurt Eggs	Beans Lentils Nuts	Iron (Energy)
Lacto vegetarian	Red meat Offal Fish Poultry Eggs	Milk Cheese Yoghurt	Beans Lentils Nuts	Iron Vitamin D (Energy)
Vegan	Red meat Offal Fish Poultry Eggs Milk Cheese Yoghurt	Beans Lentils Nuts		Iron Energy Protein Fat soluble vitamins Vitamin B_2 (Riboflavin) Vitamin B_{12} Calcium Zinc

From: Wolfe (1994) (Reproduced with permission.)

18.2.2 Vegetarian and vegan infants

Suitable milks and weaning diets are considered in Chapters 1, 2 and 6 respectively.

18.2.3 Vegetarian and vegan toddlers

It is very important that the diets of vegetarian/vegan toddlers are appropriately balanced so as to provide optimal nutrition for growth and development. The greater the restriction of animal products, the greater is the risk of nutrient deficiencies.

Vegan children are at high risk of nutrient deficiencies. Vegan parents must receive advice from a dietitian.

Use of the food group system is a helpful medium for discussing with vegetarian mothers the principles of a balanced diet (see Chapter 13). However, extra care is needed to ensure dietary adequacy in respect of some nutrients, notably energy, protein, calcium, iron and certain vitamins.

Energy
Vegetarian and vegan diets tend to be bulkier and of lower energy density than non-vegetarian diets. The energy density of vegan diets can be particularly poor due to the exclusion of dairy products. Regular assessment of the growth and development of all children on restrictive diets is an important means of monitoring energy adequacy.

What can I advise?

- Avoid giving an excessively bulky diet by limiting the use of wholegrain cereals and limiting servings of fruit and vegetables to 2–4 portions per day.
- Encourage the moderate use of oils, nut butters and ground nuts to maintain dietary energy density.

Whole nuts are not advised for young children under five years due to the risk of choking.

- Ensure a good intake of milk and dairy products, equivalent to at least 350 ml each day.
- Seek advice from a dietitian about calcium fortified soya infant milk for vegan infants.

Protein
Contrary to popular belief, many vegetable foods are good sources of protein. Examples are given in Table 18.2.

Plant sources of protein do not contain such a complete mix of amino acids as foods derived from animal sources. However, giving a

Table 18.2 Non-meat sources of protein.

Food	Examples
Milk and dairy foods	
Eggs	
Nuts	Hazelnuts, almonds, cashews (ground or in nut butter for under fives)
Seeds	Sesame, sunflower (ground or in paste, e.g. tahini, for under fives)
Pulses	Baked beans, lentils, peas
Cereals	Bread, breakfast cereal, rice, pasta
Soya products, Quorn	Tofu, textured vegetable protein, soya cheese

mixture of plant proteins will ensure that all essential amino acids are obtained. Food combinations providing 'complete' protein, i.e. all essential amino acids, include:

- Milk Products + cereals
- Milk Products + nuts
- Milk Products + pulses
- Cereals   + pulses
- Cereals   + nuts

Many of these combinations are achieved routinely. For example:

- Weetabix and milk = cereal and milk
- Beans on toast   = pulse and cereal
- Macaroni cheese   = cheese and cereal

While it is now considered unnecessary to combine protein sources at every meal (American Dietetic Association, 1993), protein sources should be mixed and a variety of foods offered at each meal. This is particularly important for vegan children.

Calcium
Vegetarian and non-vegetarian toddlers should consume a minimum of 350 ml ($\frac{2}{3}$ pint) of milk or equivalent per day to meet their calcium

requirements (see Section 13.4.1). Requirement increases after five years.

Vegan parents must use a calcium fortified soya infant milk, and require advice from a dietitian.

Calcium absorption is maximised only if vitamin D status is adequate, and vitamin D supplements, in the form of government vitamin drops, are recommended for all vegetarian and vegan children throughout the first five years.

Iron

Iron nutrition is discussed fully in Chapter 7. Iron is available from a variety of plant foods and these are important sources of iron in the diets of young children (Payne & Belton, 1992b; Mills & Tyler, 1992). Plant sources of iron include fortified breakfast cereals, bread, wholegrains such as barley, rice and oats and pulses. Dried fruit, ground nuts and nut butters, and baked goods containing them, are also useful sources. Eggs and Quorn are suitable sources of iron for vegetarian, but not vegan, children. Vitamin C rich foods should be given at the same time to maximise iron absorption from these foods (see Section 7.3.2).

Other possible nutrient deficiencies

Government vitamin drops are recommended for all vegetarian and vegan children (see above) and skin synthesis of vitamin D should be maximised by exposure to sunlight during the summer months.

A poorly constructed vegan diet risks deficiency of zinc and riboflavin and certain fatty acids, but dietary provision of these nutrients cannot be readily assessed.

Any child on a vegetarian or vegan diet with a limited dietary intake or showing poor growth requires referral to a dietitian.

Are vegetarian diets suitable for young children?

A well-balanced vegetarian/vegan diet is perfectly compatible with normal child growth and development (O'Connell *et al.*, 1989), but such diets must be constructed so as to ensure provision of all nutrients required for growth. Dietary supplements must be provided, if necessary, to compensate for any dietary restrictions. Overall, the average growth of Caucasian vegetarian children parallels that of Caucasian omnivores and, although lower rates of early growth are seen in vegan children, catch-up growth occurs by ten years (Sanders & Manning, 1992).

Highly restrictive macrobiotic-type diets, allowing minimal animal products or fats, are not suitable for young children. Nutritional deficiencies, leading to growth and developmental delay, have been widely observed with such diets.

18.3   Asian diets

18.3.1   Background

The Asian community is the largest ethnic minority in the UK. The term Asian refers generally to all people whose origins are from India, Bangladesh, Pakistan and East Africa. Dietary customs are largely based on the religious and cultural beliefs of the three main groups, Muslims, Hindus and Sikhs, but there is considerable variation in the use of foods and cooking styles within these groupings.

Some Asian communities have maintained their dietary traditions but others are increasingly influenced by westernised eating habits which often serve to reduce the quality of the diet. A summary of dietary restrictions is given in Table 18.3 and more detailed information is available in the briefing paper *Nutrition in minority ethnic groups* (HEA, 1991).

Table 18.3   Regional diets of main Asian groups in Britain.

From the Indian Punjab		From Gujarat		From Pakistan	From Bangladesh
Sikhs	**Hindus**	**Hindus**	**Muslims**	**Muslims**	**Muslims**
Main staple cereal					
chapattis	chapattis	chapattis or rice	chapattis or rice	chapattis	rice
Main fats					
ghee (clarified butter)	ghee	groundnut or mustard oil, some ghee	groundnut or mustard oil, some ghee	ghee or groundnut oil	groundnut or mustard oil, a little ghee

Continued

Table 18.3 Regional diets of main Asian groups in Britain.

From the Indian Punjab		From Gujarat		From Pakistan	From Bangladesh
Sikhs	**Hindus**	**Hindus**	**Muslims**	**Muslims**	**Muslims**
Meat and Fish					
no beef, some vegetarians, others eat mainly chicken or mutton,	no beef, mostly vegetarians	no beef, mostly vegetarians	no pork, Halal meat only (usually chicken or mutton)	no pork, Halal meat only (usually chicken or mutton)	no pork, Halal meat only (usually chicken or mutton)
no fish	no fish	no fish	little if any fish	little fish	a lot of fresh or dried fish
Eggs					
not a major part of the diet	not eaten by strict vegetarians	not eaten by strict vegetarians	usually hard-boiled, fried or omelette	usually hard-boiled, fried or omelette	few – usually hard-boiled, fried or omelette (in curries)
Dairy products					
very important milk yoghurt curd cheese	very important milk yoghurt curd cheese	important milk yoghurt	fairly important milk yoghurt	fairly important milk yoghurt	few milk
Pulses					
major source of protein	major source of protein	major source of protein	important	important	important
Vegetables and fruits					
curries, occasional salad, fresh fruit	curries, occasional salad, fresh fruit	curries, occasional salad, fresh fruit	curries, occasional salad, fresh fruit	curries, occasional salad, fresh fruit	curries, occasional salad, fresh fruit

Source: Newcastle Nutrition (1996).

18.3.2   Infant feeding practices

Bottle feeding
Studies consistently report a lower level of breastfeeding amongst
Asians in the UK than in the Caucasian population (Warrington &
Storey, 1988). Perception of bottle feeding as the western ideal, and a
lack of education promoting breastfeeding through the medium of
Asian languages, may be contributing factors.

Weaning
Both early and late weaning are common and have nutritional implications. Early weaning is often associated with excessive use of sweet
varieties of commercial weaning foods. These are the 'safest' option for
vegetarian families or families eating only Halal meat, but are low in
protein and iron. The need for suitable commercial weaning foods for
Asian families has now been recognised (DoH, 1994).

Late weaning is most common in families recently taking up
residence in the UK and can serve to delay feeding development.
Prolonged use of a feeding bottle exacerbates this tendency.

18.3.3   Common nutritional problems in early childhood

Growth
Babies born to Asian women are, on average, lighter than those born to
Caucasian women in the same area (Warrington & Storey, 1988).
Maternal undernutrition is thought to be an important contributing
factor in this. Asian infants and children appear to grow as well as
Caucasian children, but failure to thrive is not uncommon and growth
must therefore be assessed and monitored regularly.

Iron deficiency
Iron deficiency is a well-recognised problem in Asian toddlers
(Erhardt, 1986; Duggan *et al.*, 1991), especially where socio-economic
conditions are poor. Certain Asian weaning practices, such as the early
use of cow's milk as a drinking milk may contribute to poor iron
status, but lack of Asian language weaning information is also a matter
of concern. Written advice on weaning in an appropriate language
should be available for all Asian mothers.

Vitamin D deficiency and rickets
In the 1960s and 1970s rickets was found to be a significant problem in

Asian children living in urban communities. Asian children's suscept-
ibility to rickets may be increased by factors such as a diet high in
phytate and fibre (inhibiting absorption of calcium and other minerals), poor dietary intake of vitamin D and limited exposure of skin to
sunlight for cultural reasons.

Given their increased risk of deficiency, vitamin D supplementation
is recommended for Asian children throughout the first five years (see
also Section 3.4). This has been shown to reduce the incidence of
rickets in Asian children (Dunnigan *et al.*, 1985).

Dental caries

Consumption of NME sugar has become a problem within some Asian
communities and especially in young children. Practices such as adding
sugar to babies' feeding bottles at two years greatly increase risk of
early tooth decay (see Section 10.5.2). All Asian families should receive
clear dental health advice in an appropriate language.

18.4 Afro-Caribbean diets

For sources of information on traditional Afro-Caribbean foods and
diet see Resources List at the back of the book. The Afro-Caribbean
community is the second largest ethnic minority in the UK. As with the
Asian population, westernised dietary practices have become increasingly integrated with more traditional eating habits. A minority of the
Afro-Caribbean population within the UK are Rastafarians and follow
dietary laws with varying degrees of strictness. The most orthodox
Rastafarians are vegans and eat only I-tal foods. This includes exclusion of all canned food. Other Rastafarians are at nutritional risk for
reasons of social deprivation.

18.4.1 Infant feeding practices

Information on infant feeding in UK Afro-Caribbean communities is
poor, but a number of characteristic practices can be identified:

- Breastfeeding rates are high initially but drop off rapidly, and
  exclusive breastfeeding is rare
- Early weaning is common, and 45% of infants are reported to be
  receiving solid food at three months (Kemm *et al.*, 1986).
- Traditional foods (e.g. corn meal, rice, porridge) may be used for
  weaning in Rastafarian populations. These are often of low nutrient
  density.

18.4.2   Common nutritional problems

Problems encountered in Afro-Caribbean children are most commonly attributed to:

- Adverse weaning practices, or
- Unsupplemented, restrictive Rastafarian diets

Iron Deficiency Anaemia, associated with prolonged bottle feeding, late weaning and excessive use of cow's milk, has been reported (HEA, 1991). Rickets is found in Afro-Caribbean children but less commonly than in Asian children. Risk of other dietary inadequacies, such as energy and vitamin B_{12}, exists in strict Rastafarian groups.

Lactose intolerance

There is a genetic tendency to hypolactasia among the black population and hence a higher incidence of lactose intolerance than within Caucasian populations. Hypolactasia increases with age and is uncommon in infancy and early childhood.

Medical and dietetic referral is recommended for all children suspected of lactose intolerance

For more on lactose intolerance see Section 9.8.1.

18.5   Other ethnic groups

18.5.1   Chinese diets

The Chinese community is the third largest ethnic group in the UK. Very few foods are avoided but dairy products do not feature significantly in the traditional diet, therefore calcium intakes of young children should be monitored. Lactose intolerance is now more prevalent than before. Traditional diets are high in salt and advice on limiting young children's salt intake may be required.

18.5.2   Vietnamese diets

A large proportion of Vietnamese settlers in the UK are ethnic Chinese and therefore share many of the Chinese traditions. Few foods are avoided, but intake of dairy foods tends to be low; some Vietnamese children may therefore be at risk of calcium deficiency. There is also a high incidence of lactose intolerance among the Vietnamese population

(Shaw & Lawson, 1994). Deficiency of vitamin D has been noted in Vietnamese children, and government vitamin supplements are recommended for this group.

18.5.3 Jewish diets

Jewish dietary laws are based on the following principles:

(1) Food is split into three groups.
 • Milk foods – cheese, yoghurt, butter etc.
 • Meat foods – beef, lamb, poultry, meat products
 • Neutral (Parev) foods (neither meat nor milk) – fruit, vegetables, cereals, pulses
(2) Meat and milk products are not mixed at the same meal.
(3) Only Kosher meat is allowed (slaughtered according to Jewish law).
(4) Pork is not eaten.
(5) Only fish with scales and fins can be eaten, i.e. no shellfish.

As with all religious groups, families vary in their level of observance of dietary customs. Orthodox families may eat foods only from recognised Kosher sources. This can include the use of soya infant formula in preference to non-Kosher infant milk. Where dietary laws are adhered to, care must be taken to ensure that an adequate intake of dairy foods is achieved at times other than at meat-containing meals.

References and Further Reading for Section 2

American Dietetic Association (1993) Position of the ADA: vegetarian diets. *J.Am.Dietet.Assoc.*, **91**, 1317–19.

British Dietetic Association (1995) *Vegetarian Diets*: position paper. BDA, Birmingham.

Casey, P.H., Bradley, R. & Wortham, B. (1984) Social and non-social home environment of infants with non-organic failure to thrive. *Pediatrics*, **73**, 348–53.

Clayden, G.S. (1992) Management of chronic constipation. *Arch.Dis.Child.*, **67**, 340–44.

Davidson, M. & Wasserman, R. (1966) The irritable colon of childhood (chronic non-specific diarrhoea syndrome). *J. Pediatr*, **69**, 1027–38.

Davies P. & Evans, S. (1995) Diet and health in pre-school children. In *Practice Nutrition*, **4**, 2, July.

Deckelbaum, R.J. (1990) Nutrition, the child and atherosclerosis. *Acta.Paediatr.Scand.* Suppl. 365.

DoH (1991) Department of Health Dietary Reference Values for Food, Energy and Nutrients for the United Kingdom. *Report on Health and Social Subjects No. 41*. HMSO, London.

DoH (1994) Department of Health. Weaning and the Weaning Diet. *Report on Health and Social Subjects No. 45*. HMSO, London.

Duggan, M.B., Steel, G., Elwys, E., Harbo, L. & Nohle, C. (1991) Iron status, energy intake and nutritional status of healthy young Asian children. *Arch.Dis.Child.*, **66**, 1386–9.

Dunnigan, M.G., Glekin, B. M., Henderson, J.B. McIntosh, W.B., Sumner, D. & Sutherland, G.R. (1985) Prevention of rickets in Asian children: assessment of the Glasgow campaign. *B.M.J. Clinical Research Ed.*, **291**, 239–42.

Erhardt, P. (1986) Iron deficiency in young Bradford children from different ethnic groups. *B.M.J.*, **292**, 90–93

Evans, C.D.H. & Lacey, J.H. (1986) Toxicity of vitamins: complications of a health movement. *B.M.J.*, **292**, 509–10.

Francis, D. (1986) *Nutrition for Children*. Blackwell Science Ltd, Oxford.

Green, C. (1992) *Toddler Training: a Parents Guide to the First Four Years*. Vermillion, London.

Green, H.L. & Gishan, F.K. (1983) Excessive fluid intake as a cause of chronic diarrhoea in young children. *J. Pediatr.*, **102**, 836–40.

Harris B & Booth, I.W. (1992) In *Feeding Problems and Eating Disorders in Children and Adolescents* (eds P.J. Cooper & A. Stern). Harwood Academic Publishers, New York.

HEA (1991) *Nutrition in Minority Ethnic Groups.* Health Education Authority Briefing Paper. HEA, London.

Hourihane, J.O'B & Rolles, C.J. (1995) Morbidity from excessive intake of high energy fluids: the 'squash drinking' syndrome. *Arch.Dis.Child.*, 72, 141–3.

Illingworth, R.S. & Lister, J. (1964) The critical or sensitive period with special reference to certain feeding problems in infants and children. *J. Pediatr.*, 65, 839–49.

James, W.P.T., Ralph, A. & Sanchez-Castillo C.P. (1987) The dominance of salt in manufactured foods in the sodium intake of affluent societies. *Lancet*, 1, 426–9.

Kemm, J.R., Douglas, J. & Sylvester, V. (1986) A survey of infant feeding practices by Afro-Caribbean mothers in Birmingham. *Proc.Nutr.Soc.*, 45(3), 87A.

Ko, M.L.B., Ramsell, N. & Wilson, J.A. (1992) What do parents know about vitamins? *Arch.Dis.Child.*, 67, 1080–81.

Mills, A. & Tyler, H. (1992) *Food and Nutrient Intakes of British Infants, aged 6–12 months.* HMSO, London.

Minde, K. & Minde, R. (1986) *Infant Psychiatry: an Introductory Text.* Sage, London.

NCH (1991) *Poverty and Nutrition Survey.* National Children's Home, London.

Newcastle Nutrition (1996) Regional diets of main Asian groups in Britain. Personal correspondence.

O'Connell, J.M., Dibley, M.J., Sierra, J., Wallace, B., Marks, J.S. & Yip, R. (1989) Growth of vegetarian children. The Farm Study. *Pediatrics*, 84, 475–81.

Payne, J.A. & Belton, N.R. (1992a) Nutrient intake and growth in pre-school children I. Comparison of energy intake and sources of energy with growth. *J.Hum.Nutr.Dietet.*, 5, 15–26.

Payne, J.A. & Belton, N.R. (1992b) Nutrient intake and growth in pre-school children II. Intake of minerals and vitamins. *J.Hum.Nutr.Dietet.*, 5, 27–32.

Rose, G., Stamler, R., Elliott, P., Dyer, A. & Marmot, M. (1989) Intersalt study findings – public health and medical care implications. *Hypertension*, 14, 570–77.

Sanders, T. & Manning, J. (1992) The growth and development of vegan children. *J.Hum.Nutr.Dietet.*, 5, 11–12.

Scottish Office (1993) *The Scottish Diet*: report of a working party to the Chief Medical Officer for Scotland. Scottish Home and Health Department, Edinburgh.

Shaw, V. & Lawson, M. (eds) (1994) *Clinical Paediatric Dietetics*. Blackwell Science Ltd, Oxford.

Skuse, D. (1993) Identification and management of problem eaters. *Arch. Dis.Child.*, **69**, 604–8.

Southern Derbyshire Health Authority (1993) *Infant Feeding Policy for Health Professionals, 'Feeding, The Right Advice'*. Southern Derbyshire Health Authority and Derbyshire Family Health Services Authority.

Stordy, B.J. (1994) Is it appropriate to apply adult healthy eating guidelines to babies and young children? In *The Growing Cycle*, proceedings of a conference. National Dairy Council, London.

Taitz,. L.S. (1987) Diet of young children and cardiovascular disease. *B.M.J.*, **294**, 920–21.

Taitz L.S. & Wardley, B.L. (1990) *Handbook of Child Nutrition*. Oxford University Press, Oxford.

Walker, C. & Cannon, G. (1984) *The Food Scandal*. Century Publishing, London.

Walker-Smith, J. (1980) Toddlers' diarrhoea. *Arch.Dis.Child.*, **55**, 329–30.

Walker-Smith, J. (1987) Commentary on gastrointestinal food allergy in childhood. In *Food Intolerance* (ed. J. Dobbing). Ballière Tindall, London.

Warrington, S. & Storey, D.M. (1988) Comparative studies on Asian and Caucasian children. 2: Nutrition feeding practices and health. *Eur. J.Clin.Nutr.*, **42**, 69–80.

Wolfe, S. (1994) Children from ethnic minorities and those following cultural diets. In *Clinical Paediatric Dietetics* (eds V. Shaw & M. Lawson). Blackwell Science Ltd, Oxford.

Further reading

ILEA (1985) *Inner London Education Authority Nutritional Guidelines*. ILEA, London.

Milla, P.J. (1991) The clinical use of protein hydrolysates and soya formulae. *Eur.J.Clin.Nutr.*, **45** (Suppl.1) 23–8.

Whiting, M. & Lobstein, T. (1992) *The Nursery Food Book*. London Food Commission, London.

Section 3
Three to Five Years

19. The Healthy Pre-school Diet

> 'One of the first principles of healthy eating is that the requirement for the essential nutrients must be met.'
>
> Thomas, 1994

This chapter covers:

- The nutrient needs of pre-school children
- How nutrient needs can be met
- The importance of regular meals
- Suitable snacks

The period from 1–3 years has been described as the initial phase of dietary transition from infant to adult-style eating habits. This process continues from 3–5 years and the term pre-school is used to describe this stage. The pre-school period is characterised by a slowed rate of growth, relative body leanness and increasing developmental skills and independence. These factors affect both nutrient needs and food intake. From the age of three years, a child's food preferences and eating habits are also increasingly influenced by factors outside the home. Nursery school, peer group preference, television advertising and experience of eating away from home can all be determinants of food choices.

The pre-school diet must therefore not only meet nutritional needs for growth, body repair and daily activity, but also reinforce good eating habits and seek to respond to the challenges of potentially adverse influences.

19.1 Nutrient needs

The nutrient needs of pre-school children are not readily defined because young children vary widely in their energy and nutrient intakes and requirements. Dietary reference value (DRV) figures are a guide to average nutrient requirements but cannot be used to determine the nutrient needs of an individual child. DRV values are given in Appendix II.

How can nutrient needs be met?

As with toddlers, nutrient needs are most likely to be met if a **variety** of different foods is eaten from each of the four main food groups every day (see Chapter 13 – Assessing Dietary Adequacy). The number of servings advised is shown in Table 19.1. Appetite should be allowed to determine an increased intake of bread or cereals if required. As with toddlers, sweet foods and drinks should be limited to meal times.

Table 19.1 Advised number of servings.

Food groups	Number of servings each day
Meat, fish and alternatives	2
Milk and dairy foods	3
Bread, other cereals and potatoes	4 +
Fruit and vegetables	2 fruits and 2 vegetables
Fatty and sugary	2 Moderate amount of margarine or butter

Specific nutrient needs

Detailed information on the function of different nutrients is given in Chapter 6 – Weaning, and Chapter 12 – Nutritional Requirements 1–3 Years.

Energy

Requirements are increased in accordance with age, but are **lower** in relation to kg body weight. This reflects lower growth rate. Daily energy intakes are often highly variable in pre-school children and weight gain normally fluctuates. Regular monitoring of weight and height long-term is the best means of assessing whether energy intake is adequate.

Protein

The protein requirement of the pre-school child is the same as that of the toddler, i.e. 1.1 g protein per kg body weight. Parents can be reassured that protein deficiency is rare in the UK. Even young children with otherwise poor diets generally achieve protein adequacy (Payne & Belton, 1992a).

Calcium

The calcium requirement of children aged 4–6 years is greater than that of younger children. Milk and dairy products are therefore an important part of the pre-school diet. Semi-skimmed milk, which contains as much calcium as whole milk, can be given to pre-school children, provided energy intake is adequate.

Iron

Iron requirement from 4–6 years is less than that from 1–3 years, but low iron status has been noted in pre-school children of all ages (Gregory *et al.*, 1995). The incidence of low iron status declines with increasing age, but all pre-school children require a daily intake of iron rich foods, together with vitamin C rich foods, to promote iron absorption.

Vitamins

Requirements for B vitamins increase from 4–6 years but requirement is usually met by the general increase in food consumption. Low intakes of vitamin C have been observed in young children (Payne & Belton, 1992b), but the 1995 survey of pre-school children's nutrient intakes (Gregory *et al.*, 1995) found vitamin C intakes to be satisfactory. Vitamin D status was considered to be more of a problem. As a safeguard supplementary vitamin drops, supplying vitamins A, D and C, are recommended for all young children from 1–5 years. This is particularly important for 'at risk' groups such as Asian/Afro–Caribbean children, poor eaters and children on restricted diets.

19.2   Healthy eating habits

Eating **habits** encompass both **what** is eaten (food choice) and **how** it is eaten (eating pattern).

Food choices

The healthy pre-school diet should comprise a varied daily intake of different foods from each of the food groups. Consumption of sugary and fatty foods should be limited and a moderate intake of fibre from both vegetables and fruit and cereal sources is to be encouraged (see Chapter 14 – Eating for Future Health).

Eating patterns

Good pre-school eating patterns are equally important because they influence energy and nutrient intake, and dental health. An optimum eating pattern is generally agreed to comprise:

(1)   Regular meals
(2)   Low sugar, nutritious snacks
(3)   Low fat, nutritious snacks

19.2.1   Regular meals

What is meant by the term meal?
The *Oxford Dictionary of Current English* defines meal as: 'occasion when food is eaten'. The term meal is often understood to mean a cooked meal with vegetables, but breakfast cereal, milk and orange juice, or a cheese and tomato sandwich with a glass of milk is just as much a meal as shepherd's pie and peas. A meal is therefore any significant contribution to daily nutrient intake.

Why are regular meals important?

- Young children have small appetites but large nutrient needs relative to their body size. Regular 'refuelling' is therefore required.
- Traditionally spaced meals encourage a varied intake of foods from each of the food groups. It is harder to achieve nutritional adequacy if snacking throughout the day is the norm.
- Meal times provide a day with structure and routine, important for young children.
- Regular meals promote regular bowel habits.
- Distinct meal times, with only limited between-meal snacks, allow the child to learn about feeling hungry and feeling full. An eating pattern built on intermittent snacking does not allow this difference to be learned and may encourage a calorie intake in excess of need.
- An eating pattern based on distinct meals promotes dental health. When time is allowed to elapse between eating events, mouth acid can be neutralised efficiently by saliva and risk of dental decay is lessened.
- Meals allow opportunity for socialising and for parents to set a good example in respect of food choices and eating behaviour.

Family meal patterns are inevitably affected by family routines, parents' working hours and the child's appetite at different times of day. None of these factors should prevent a regular meal pattern being established.

So what can I advise about meals?
Highlight the nutritional and social advantages of regular meals, emphasise the benefits of routine to a child and explain that 'meal' need not mean 'cooked meal'.

19.2.2   Selective snacks

The term snack has increasingly come to be associated with foods of low nutritional value – e.g. crisps, potato snacks, chips, chocolate – but the *Oxford Dictionary of Current English* defines snack as 'Light, casual or hurried meal', or 'small amount of food eaten between meals'.

A snack should therefore be a nutritious mini-meal. Sharing snacks can be an important means of social interaction for young children and this approach to eating can sometimes encourage food refusers.

However, there are suitable and not so suitable snacks. Snacks high in non-milk extrinsic sugars (NMEs) greatly increase risk of dental caries, and an excessive intake of high fat, high sugar snacks will lead to an energy intake in excess of need. Too many snacks will reduce appetite for meals, often to the detriment of total nutrient intake.

What is a suitable snack?
One which:

- Provides nutrients other than calories
- Is low in NMEs
- Does not interfere with appetite for meals

Practical factors also need to be taken into account. Suitable snacks must therefore be readily available, affordable and appealing to a child.

Best snacks are those chosen from the **Bread and cereals** or **Fruit and vegetables** food groups. Examples include bread roll, toast, plain cracker, oatcake, banana, satsuma. These comply with the criteria listed above. A comprehensive list of snacks is given in Section 23.3.

Barriers to healthy snack habits

- Television marketing of less healthy snacks

- Peer group's influence over food preference
- Long-standing family taste preferences
- Nursery school and child care snack choices
- Greater availability of less healthy snacks

Changing established eating habits is notoriously difficult. Parents need to recognise the importance of encouraging and setting an appropriate example of good snack habits.

19.3   Eating patterns and dental health

Dental caries is prevalent in pre-school children yet it is largely preventable. As described in Chapter 10, the incidence of dental caries is directly related to the amount of NME sugars in the diet (Holt, 1990).

Frequent NME sugars + mouth bacteria → acid → demineralisation of enamel = risk of decay

Given that the risk of caries is also affected by the *frequency* of NME sugar consumption, eating patterns can exert a significant influence on dental health. When sugars are restricted to meal times only, there is a diluting effect exerted by other foods on the acid produced by mouth bacteria. Additionally, chewing stimulates saliva production, and with the benefit of time, mouth pH is raised between eating episodes, thereby preventing demineralisation (Fig. 19.1).

When the time interval between sugar consumption is short, as in the case of 'sweetie grazing', the risk of decay is high (Fig. 19.1). Thus:

Frequent NME sugars + mouth bacteria → frequent acid → prolonged demineralisation = high risk of decay

What can I advise about eating patterns and dental health?

- Keep foods and drinks containing NME sugars for meal times
- Allow time between eating episodes (so that saliva can buffer mouth acid effectively)
- Do not give fruit juice, sugary drinks or fizzy drinks over prolonged periods
- Do not give sugary drinks or snacks 'to go to bed with'.

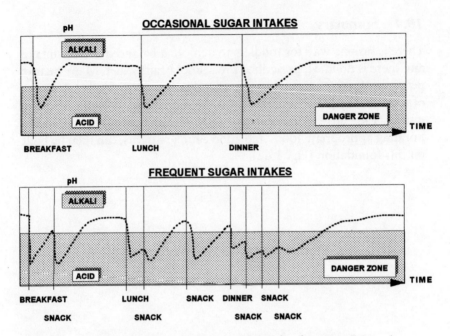

Fig. 19.1 Effect of eating patterns on the risk of caries. *From: A Handbook of Dental Health for Health visitors* (HEA, 1992).

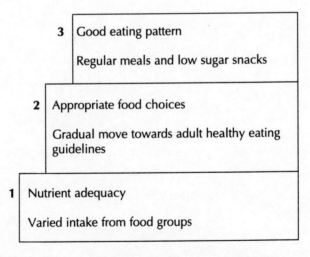

Fig. 19.2 Three steps to the healthy pre-school diet.

19.4   Summary

There is no one way for toddlers to achieve a balanced dietary intake and there is no ideal, prescribed pre-school healthy diet. Many factors determine food provision by parents and influence the food preferences of a child. The pre-school diet must, before all else, provide adequate nutrients for growth and energy needs. Healthy eating habits, incorporating appropriate foods and good eating patterns, can then be built on this foundation (Fig. 19.2).

20. Poverty and Nutrition

> 'Lack of money not ignorance is the reason for poor diet.'
>
> NCH, 1991

This chapter covers:

- The impact of low income on diet
- The link between low income and poor diet
- Possible outcomes of a poor quality diet in childhood
- Practical advice on low cost nutritious food for children

Poverty has a direct impact on the quality of children's food intake and several major studies have highlighted this relationship (NCH, 1991; Gregory *et al.*, 1995).

Set against the standards of a healthy diet (Scottish Office, 1993; DoH, 1994), it is clear that families with the lowest incomes have the poorest diet. Families on low incomes have to spend a disproportionate amount of their income on food. The NCH (1991) survey found that low income families spent around 35% of their income on food, compared with an average family expenditure of 15%.

Significantly, poverty has been defined as 'the need to spend more than 30% of income on food'.

20.1 Characteristics of low income diet

The diets of low income families should not be prejudged since some families eat diets which are well in line with current healthy eating guidelines and set an inspiring example (Lawrence, 1991). Many families, however, do not have a balanced intake and the diet of many low income families is characterised by:

- Few fruits and vegetables (except potatoes)
- Cereal and starchy foods of low fibre content
- Low quality meat products and little lean meat
- Variable servings of dairy products
- Significant amounts of fatty and sugary foods
- Limited variety

What are the nutritional implications of a poor quality diet?
A poor quality diet risks:

- Impaired growth
- Developmental delay
- Poor vitamin and mineral status
- Dental disease

In essence, low birth weight, short stature, iron deficiency and dental disease are all conditions more prevalent in children of disadvantaged families. In adult life, low income groups show consistently higher rates of diet-related diseases such as coronary heart disease (CHD), stomach cancer, obesity and hypertension, than other income groups; and many of the degenerative processes involved may start in childhood with poor dietary habits and poor quality diet.

20.2   Constraints to healthy eating

Healthy eating can appear an almost unattainable goal for low income families. Parents on low incomes are, generally, aware of the link between diet and health and know what constitutes a healthy diet (NCH, 1991). For many there are major barriers to achieving a healthy diet, including:

- Cost of healthier foods
- Availability of healthier foods
- Inadequate cooking and food storage facilities
- Limited cooking skills

20.2.1   Cost

Cost is the overriding constraint to a healthier diet for low income families (NCH, 1991). Income Support payments are currently based on the concept of 'minimum expenditure below which good health cannot be sustained' (Nelson & Peploe, 1990). Income at this level has been shown to enable the purchase of adequate quantities of nutrients, but *not* a diet in line with current healthy eating guidelines (Mooney, 1990). A healthy diet is therefore out of the financial reach of many low income families.

A number of studies have examined the cost differences between a basket of healthy and less healthy foods and have found healthy baskets to be between 13–40% more expensive than less healthy baskets (Cole-Hamilton & Lang, 1986; Hollington & Newby, 1995).

Savings made on buying fewer sugary foods and fats *do not* compensate for the increased cost of buying leaner meat, lower fat dairy products, more bread, cereals, fruit and vegetables. Fat and sugar are cheap sources of calories. Purchase of cheap, calorie dense foods enables adequate intake of most nutrients in a form acceptable to children. This is well-illustrated by considering snack food costs (Table 20.1). In addition to this, healthy foods bought in deprived areas commonly cost more than the same foods bought in affluent areas (Sooman & Taggart, 1992).

Table 20.1   Cost of 100 kilocalories of various snack foods.

Food item	Amount	Cost pence
Custard cream biscuit	2 biscuits	5.1
Ice cream	1 scoop	7.5
Chocolate bar	$\frac{1}{2}$ bar	10.0
Crisps (multi-pack)	$\frac{2}{3}$ bag	10.0
Banana	1 medium	14.0
Apple	3 small	21.9
Orange	2 medium	36.2

Adapted from: data collated by The Food Commission (1996).

A healthy diet can cost the same as one which is less healthy but only if a high proportion of income is already spent on food (NCH, 1991) or if a family is resourceful, committed, has some knowledge of cookery and access to adequate kitchen facilities.

What hidden costs need to be considered?
The costs of transport to shops and of cooking need to be taken into account. Access to cheaper foods is a major problem for many families. Travel costs can make supermarket shopping as expensive as buying food in smaller shops. Supermarket shopping also risks additional expenditure resulting from purchases of non-essential food items. Even the cost of cooking can appear prohibitive. Cooking one meal per day is estimated to cost between £1.45 and £2.15 per week, and some healthy foods (e.g. oven baked potatoes) may require longer cooking time than less healthy choices.

20.2.2   Availability

Foods considered to be healthy are often less readily available in deprived areas than affluent areas (Mooney, 1990). The range of foods stocked by shops is often limited and supermarkets in socially deprived areas tend to offer a poorer range of goods than in other areas.

Food co-operatives, offering healthy foods at reasonable prices, are one solution to this problem. They are well-established in some areas such as Bolton and Glasgow, but more are needed.

20.2.3   Cooking and food storage facilities

Achieving a varied and healthy diet is extremely difficult without access to a cooker or refrigerator.

20.2.4   Cooking skills

Basic ingredients such as raw minced beef and vegetables are cheaper than processed alternatives, but require preparation. A lack of basic cooking skills is a recognised problem in low income groups (James, 1992). This may be the result of limited early experience of cooking combined with a lack of motivation to learn. Depression and low self-esteem is not uncommon among mothers on a low income, and depression is a major barrier to change. There may also be reluctance to try new recipes in case they are rejected and the food wasted.

20.3   Tackling common problems

Health professionals can do little to alleviate the financial situation of low income families, and for many families this is the single factor most likely to improve nutritional status. Dietary improvements can enhance the health and educational development of children from low income families. Advice can usefully be targeted towards three goals:

(1)   Increasing intake of iron-rich foods
(2)   Increasing intake of fruit and vegetables
(3)   Reducing sugar intake

20.3.1   Increasing iron intake

Children from low income families are at increased risk of iron deficiency. Reasons include:

- A low intake of more expensive foods such as beef and lamb, which provide iron of high bioavailability (haem iron)
- An insufficient or poorly targeted intake of vitamin C rich foods, preventing maximum absorption of non-haem iron from plant foods
- Less structured meal patterns limiting the opportunity for consumption of iron-rich foods

What practical advice can I give?

(1) *Buy economical sources of haem iron*
Some cheaper meats are rich in iron: liver, beefburger, corned beef, minced beef (drained of fat), tinned fish (sardines, pilchards etc.).

(2) *Extend meat with pulses or vegetables*
This reduces the cost and can provide non-haem iron and vitamin C. As examples:

- Tinned burger bites/sausages and beans
- Lentils/kidney beans + minced beef
- Corned beef + baked beans
- Stew or casserole + vegetables

(3) *Give plenty of foods containing non-haem iron*
Iron fortified breakfast cereals are the cheapest source of iron in the diet (Lawson, 1994). Other cost-effective sources include bread, baked beans, tinned peas, frozen peas, raisins and malt loaf. Eggs and broccoli are useful sources of iron, but more expensive.

(4) *Give vitamin C rich foods at mealtimes*
This will maximise iron absorption. Cheapest sources of vitamin C (Lawson, 1994):

- Unsweetened orange juice
- Green cabbage
- Potato
- Instant mashed potato
- Vitamin C enriched diluting fruit drink

Other good sources are whole citrus fruits and kiwi fruit.

(5) *Limit* tea, coffee and cola drinks so that iron availability is maximised.

(6) *Give chocolate only at mealtimes*
     Chocolate is not a recommended food, but it is a significant
     source of iron in many children's diets. If chocolate is given,
     recommend that it is given at a meal. This is potentially less
     harmful to teeth and will maximise iron absorption.

20.3.2   Increasing fruit and vegetable intake

Many low income families eat little fruit and vegetables. Fruit and
vegetables are generally perceived as an expensive source of calories
and therefore to be purchased only infrequently. However, fruit and
vegetables can be a cost-effective source of vitamins and minerals.
Eating more fruit and vegetables would greatly improve the quality of
the diets of many children of low income families, as illustrated in
Table 20.2.

Table 20.2   Possible benefits of a daily fruit and vegetable intake.

Change	Effect
Increase vitamin C status	Improved iron absorption Increased efficiency of immune system Improved antioxidant vitamin status
Increase antioxidant status	Protective effect on long-term health
Increase fibre intake	Resolve tendency to constipation Promote long-term bowel health
Reduce intake of NME sugars	Improved dental health
Increase intake of minerals, e.g. calcium, iron	Build body stores

What practical advice can I give?

(1) *Buy 'value for money' vegetables*
     - Good vitamin value for money: cabbage, carrots, potato,
       instant mashed potato, tinned peas, baked beans, tinned
       tomato, swede, parsnip, broccoli
     - Frozen vegetables have a high vitamin content but can be
       expensive
     - Tinned vegetables
     - Buy fresh vegetables in season.

(2) *Buy 'value for money' fruit*
- Good vitamin value for money: bananas, kiwi fruit, satsuma, orange, raisins
- Fruits for cooking: apples, rhubarb; a small amount can go further than fresh fruit
- Tinned fruit, preferably in unsweetened juice; good buys: pineapple, peaches, mandarin segments, pears

20.3.3 Reducing sugar intake

Frequent intake of NME sugars is associated with a high risk of dental caries and caries is more likely in low income families (Holt *et al.*, 1988; Evans & Dowell, 1991).

Why do families have such high sugar intakes?

- A cheap source of calories
- Readily acceptable to children so risk of wastage is minimal
- An affordable treat
- Readily available and heavily marketed

Other more complex factors may also be involved. Cooked meals are eaten less than daily in many low income families and this can lead to an increased intake of sweet snacks. Sugary juice drinks containing vitamin C may be given as a cheap source of vitamin C, in the belief that they are of benefit. The impact of high sugar intake is often exacerbated by lack of, or irregular, tooth brushing and dental visits.

What practical advice can I give?

- Reduce the frequency with which sweet foods and drinks are given
- Remember that giving sweet foods at meal times is acceptable but frequent sugary snacks or drinks will greatly increase the risk of tooth decay
- Give low sugar snacks (see Table 20.3). These can be as low cost as sweet alternatives (see Table 20.1).
- Give non-sweet drinks between meals (see Section 23.4).

Further suggestions on reducing sugar intake are given in Section 14.3. Advice to reduce sugar intake should include:

- Daily supervised tooth brushing
- Use of fluoride toothpaste

Table 20.3 Costed low sugar snacks.

Snack	Cost to nearest 1p
1 slice of bread	4
1 bread roll	9
1 slice of bread + fish paste	11
1 slice of bread + smooth peanut butter	8
1 slice of bread + scraping of Marmite	13
1 oatcake	8
2 crackers	5
2 crackers + cheese spread	8
2 bread sticks	10
1 plain biscuit (e.g. tea biscuit)	1
1 drop scone	15
1 fruit scone	11
Small bowl of plain cereal with milk	19
Cup of milk (150 ml)	7
Cheese triangle	9
Carrot (medium)	4
Banana (small)	11
Apple	15
Satsuma	9
Kiwi fruit	19
Handful of raisins (30 g)*	7

From: supermarket, 1997 prices

* Dried fruit is a concentrated source of sugar. Tooth brushing, or at least a drink of water, is recommended after eating dried fruit.

- Registration with a dentist
- Regular dental check-ups

All dental advice and treatment is free for children. Any child considered to be in need of specialist advice should be referred to the community dental service.

20.4 Summary

The nutritional problems experienced by children of low income families reflect those of all pre-school children but occur with increased frequency. Providing a healthy diet for children can take considerable commitment and motivation on the part of parents. This level of motivation may, for many reasons, be difficult to sustain for low income families. Dietary change can make a significant improvement to the health of children from low income families, but advice must be directed at economically viable change.

21. Feeding Problems

> 'An infinite variety of food combinations can provide an adequate diet'
>
> Francis, 1987

This chapter covers:

- Causes of food fads
- Factors influencing a child's food preferences
- Practical advice to parents of faddy eaters

21.1 Food fads

Many young children pass through a phase of being faddy about food and refusing to eat certain foods. Faddiness exists in varying degrees, but at its most extreme, the diet can appear quite bizarre. The apparent lack of dietary variety resulting from faddy eating can be a source of considerable anxiety to parents, but food faddiness will be resolved naturally if allowed to and rarely has an adverse effect on the child's health.

What causes food fads?
Food faddiness, like food refusal, is psychologically based and often has many underlying causes. It is commonly used as an attention seeking device and the behaviour is often reinforced by parents' anxiety. Much of the discussion concerning the causes of food refusal are relevant to food faddiness (see Section 16.1).

21.1.1 Food likes and dislikes

Food faddiness tends to reflect the extremes of young children's food likes and dislikes. Food likes and dislikes, in turn, are influenced by:

- Taste
- Familiarity
- Parents' or carers' food preferences
- Parents' or carers' attitudes to food
- Food appeal

Consideration of these factors promotes understanding of the origins of food fads.

Taste

Taste is an important factor in determining food choice throughout life; taste sensitivity is affected by a number of physiological factors, including genetics. Bitter compounds are present in foods commonly rejected by children, e.g. turnip, broccoli, green beans. Initial aversion may be overcome but individuals with low thresholds for bitter tastes do appear to have more food dislikes than those with higher thresholds (Fischer *et al.*, 1961).

Familiarity

Most young children thrive on routine and are more content and happy when they live in a structured environment. Familiar foods, like familiar routines, can provide security and this may contribute to the reluctance of many toddlers to try new tastes. In evolutionary terms avoidance of unfamiliar foods enhances a child's chances of survival (Skuse, 1993). Exposure to a wide variety of tastes during infancy is the easiest means of achieving a varied intake in the pre-school years, but if this stage is 'missed', repeated exposure to a food does increase familiarity and thereby acceptability (Finney, 1986).

Parents'/others' food preferences

Young children are extremely unlikely to eat a wide range of foods unless their parents, siblings and other people around them do so. Social contact and interaction is a powerful influence on food likes and dislikes. Young children commonly reject food which they have seen others rejecting, and may demand foods which they have seen others eating. The strong influence of peer group over food preference is widely seen in nursery school children.

Parents'/others' attitudes to foods

Adults find it extremely difficult to be objective about food. The foods which children tend to dislike are often those which parents think are 'good' or 'healthy', but the pressure to eat such foods is a strong incentive to the child *not* to eat them. Similarly, foods which are presented as treats and rewards come to hold high status. Bribing a child to eat a disliked food negatively influences the child's preference for that food, i.e. bribery to eat is counter-productive.

Food appeal

The shape, flavour and colour of foods exert a strong influence on children's food choice. Food needs to be interesting to look at (in colour and shape), non-threatening and not bitter-tasting. The importance of initial food appeal is well recognised by food manufacturers who spend huge sums of money promoting their products to young children: yoghurt pots with feet, character pasta shapes, chocolate breakfast cereals.

Does food faddiness matter?

Food faddiness matters in so far as it can be a social disadvantage but it rarely has an adverse effect on a child's nutritional status. Many parents worry that the lack of dietary variety associated with food faddiness will result in an inadequate nutrient intake, but such fears are unfounded. Eating a variety of different foods at each meal is desirable but it is not essential, and a varied diet can be achieved in the space of a day or even a week.

Variety can also mean the *same* variety each day, such as when children restrict their intake to just a few different foods. In these cases, the foods selected do often make up a reasonably balanced intake. An example of this would be a chosen diet of Weetabix, baked beans and banana. Eating a wide variety of foods is, of course, preferable, but given time and encouragement it is almost always possible to increase dietary variety eventually.

21.1.2 Management of food fads

As with food refusal, the key to management of food fads is reassuring parents in respect of their child's health and minimising the manipulative effect of the behaviour. Refusal of specific types of food – e.g. meat, vegetables – is often of particular concern to parents and therefore considered separately.

General points

In all cases, a child's weight and height should be measured and plotted on the appropriate centile chart in order to assess growth adequacy. In the majority of cases the parents can then be reassured accordingly. If growth is poor, the child should be referred for medical and dietary assessment.

Management plan

The following is a detailed plan for discussion with well-motivated parents. Many of the suggestions relating to the management of food refusal are relevant (see Section 16.1).

(1) List all foods and drinks the child *will* eat. (This can help to reassure parents in respect of dietary variety).

(2) If milk or juice is drunk in excessive quantities, limit intake to about three cups per day.

(3) From the 'will eat' list, serve one choice of food at each meal. *Do not* offer an alternative if this is rejected.

(4) Continue to serve the child foods that the rest of the family are eating, but in tiny quantities, e.g. two peas, 1 tsp mince. Encourage the child to taste the food, but *do not* insist that it is eaten.

(5) Praise highly when any new food is eaten.

(6) Invite the child to serve himself as much as possible.

(7) Be seen to eat a wide range of foods and enjoy them.

(8) Avoid describing foods as good or bad.

(9) Do not force, coax or cajole the child to eat.

(10) Do not react to food left uneaten.

(11) Limit meal times to 20 minutes.

(12) Do not give between-meal snacks other than perhaps a piece of fruit or plain cracker.

(13) Encourage the child to help with food related activities such as shopping and meal preparation.

(14) Allow plenty of opportunity for social eating.

Management of individual children varies greatly according to parents' level of anxiety, degree of faddiness, home circumstances etc., but consistency is central to successful management of food fads; parents need to establish management 'rules' and stick to them.

21.2 Refusal to eat meat

Meat is not an essential component of a young child's diet, but it is a good source of many essential nutrients. Young children often show a disinclination to eat lumps of meat, but will accept it in other forms.

What can I advise?

• Try giving meat in less recognisable forms, e.g. beefburger, sausage, corned beef hash.

- Serve tiny portions of meat with known favourite tastes, e.g. diced ham in macaroni cheese, mince with tomato ketchup.
- Try different kinds of chicken and fish dishes: minced or mashed in rissoles, fish cakes.
- Try a few meatless meals using eggs, cheese, beans. Occasional use of commercial products saves preparation time.
- Give plenty of other iron-containing foods, e.g. fortified breakfast cereal, green vegetables as well as vitamin C-containing fruit and vegetables to enhance iron absorption.
- Continue to offer small tastes of different kinds of meat and meat products. Familiarity promotes acceptance.

21.3   Refusal to eat vegetables

Vegetables, especially green varieties, are often rejected. Some vegetables do appear bitter to young children, but equally parents can exert a negative influence on child's tastes, i.e. by overcooking vegetables so that they are sludge green in colour, force feeding because of their inherent 'good for you' image and serving too large portions. It is important to remember that vegetables come in many forms. It is very rare for a young child to refuse all vegetables.

What can I advise?

- Give the recommended dose of five government vitamin drops daily to ensure that requirements for vitamins A and C are met.
- Avoid giving greens for a while. Give reds, oranges and yellows instead – for example, carrots, tomatoes, sweet potato, sweetcorn. Many of these vegetables are naturally sweet.
- Serve vegetables raw instead of cooked and in pieces which can be eaten with fingers.
- Use vegetables disguised as purées in soups and sauces.
- Allow the child to serve himself.
- Present vegetables in a positive light and be seen to be eating them.
- Make the most of vegetables as the focus of games, for example:
  o Washing vegetables
  o Making salad
  o Potato printing
  o Growing cress
  o Sprouting carrot tops

21.4   Refusal to drink milk

Refusal to drink milk is not uncommon, but milk is often acceptable in other forms, e.g. cheese or yoghurt. Encourage these foods daily as well as a good intake of other sources of calcium-containing foods (see Section 13.4.1). Refer for dietary assessment if intake of all milk products continues to be poor.

21.5   Summary

Food faddiness is a common form of childhood food refusal and often reflects the extremes of a child's food preferences. Faddiness rarely affects a child's nutritional status since even very limited diets can meet nutrient requirements. Management of food fads depends on minimising the disruptive effect of a child's behaviour and alleviating parental anxiety. Food faddiness almost always recovers by itself when allowed to do so.

22. Obesity

'Obesity is the commonest nutritional disorder in Britain.'

Francis, 1987

This chapter covers:

- The causes of excessive childhood weight gain
- Practical advice on reducing energy intake

22.1 Definitions

Obesity can be defined as:

'The condition in which there is excess accumulation of adipose fat, resulting from excess energy intake over expenditure.'

(Garrow, 1978)

or

'... an excess of adipose tissue, considered to be undesirable or to reach levels above those set arbitrarily and based on a suitable anthropometric measurement.'

(Taitz, 1991)

22.2 Assessment

There are no agreed criteria to assess relative fatness in children. Weight and height measurements should be plotted on centile charts. Weight alone cannot be used to determine obesity since a heavy child is not necessarily an overweight child. Height must always be taken into account. In general, a weight of more than two centiles higher than height constitutes obesity (Shaw & Lawson, 1994).

What other assessments can be made?
In adults, calculation of body mass index (BMI) using the equation weight (kg) divided by height (m^2), gives an indication of the degree of obesity. In children, BMI calculations must be used with reference

charts. These have recently been published (Cole *et al.*, 1995) and national charts are available from the Child Growth Foundation. BMI scores may help to identify children at risk of becoming obese (Rolland-Cachera *et al.*, 1984; White *et al.*, 1995).

Measurement of skinfold thickness is rarely undertaken, but it gives a true indication of fatness and can be compared with centile chart data. In practice, obesity is commonly defined by appearance: a child is obese if he looks fat.

22.3 Adiposity during childhood

Parents need to appreciate that children's rate of weight gain and degree of fatness is different at different ages. During the first six months of life body weight doubles and body fat trebles. This accumulation of fat is thought to be of evolutionary advantage in preparation for weaning.

Will a chubby infant become an overweight adult?
There is little correlation between infant and adult obesity, i.e. the 'overweight' infant does not necessarily become an overweight adult (Poskitt, 1991) and an infant who is chubby at one year is likely to slim down as mobility increases.

What about overweight toddlers and young children?
Weight gain in the lean post-toddler period (2–6 years) is thought to be of some significance in determining later obesity and is therefore to be avoided. Adult obesity is *not* an inevitable result of childhood obesity, but it is known that obese children have a greater risk of becoming obese adults than non-obese children (Serdula *et al.*, 1993).

22.4 Causes of obesity

What makes a child overweight?
Obesity results from an interaction of genetic, environmental and psychological factors. Psychological factors are also a major determinant of eating behaviour.

22.4.1 Genetic factors

Many studies support the theory that obesity tends to run in families. The risk of a child becoming overweight is greatly increased if:

- Both parents are overweight
- Other siblings are overweight

Genetic factors are thought to determine relative vulnerability to weight gain, which is then influenced by environmental factors.

22.4.2   Environmental factors

Eating habits and lifestyle play a significant part in the development of obesity. Contributory factors include:

- A bad example set by parents regarding the type and amount of food bought and consumed
- A high intake of fatty and sugary foods
- Preference for snacking and eating on the move
- Reduced physical activity in favour of sedentary entertainments

These factors serve to increase energy intake and decrease energy expenditure. They are often inter-related. Consumption of high fat, high sugar snacks is greater where meal pattern is poor. Sedentary activities, e.g. computer games, involve little energy expenditure and encourage snacking behaviour. Some overweight parents exert a major influence over early eating habits but often eat poorly themselves.

Some environmental factors determining risk of obesity cannot be modified, e.g. social class. Social class is inversely related to prevalence of obesity and children of lower social class are more likely to become obese (RCP, 1983).

22.4.3   Psychological factors

Psychological reasons for over-eating serve to highlight the emotional significance of food to both young children and adults caring for them. A child can learn to associate food with emotions and behaviours. This may result from:

- Parents use of food as a substitute for affection or attention
- Use of food to reward, provide a treat, bribe or comfort
- Parents tendency to feed-up their children by encouraging the finishing of all meals; this can result in children being unable to determine their own satiety level
- A child's desire to please parents by finishing meals

- Comfort eating due to boredom, emotional distress or insecurity
- Eating in front of the television

22.5   Consequences of childhood obesity

The need to prevent and treat childhood obesity is generally related to its persistence into adulthood and the subsequent increased risk of hypertension, hyperlipidaemia and diabetes. These conditions are all recognised risk factors for coronary heart disease and cerebrovascular disease.

The most prevalent consequences of childhood obesity are psycho-social. Teasing is commonplace and serves to undermine self-esteem and isolate the overweight child from its peer group. The resulting insecurity and isolation may predispose to comfort eating or difficult behaviour. In addition, being overweight can act as a major disin-centive to participate in physical activity and this exacerbates the problem of obesity.

22.6   Prevention of obesity

Preventing a child from becoming overweight is infinitely preferable to tackling the problem when it arises. Given the interaction between genetic and environmental factors in the aetiology of obesity, it is to some degree possible to identify children at risk of becoming over-weight.

Risk factors for obesity

- One or more overweight parents
- Overweight siblings
- Family diet known to be inappropriate
- Low income family

Where the family diet is considered to be inappropriate, dietary modification to reduce fat and total energy intake is advisable (see below) but childhood obesity cannot be prevented without parents' co-operation.

22.7   Management of early childhood obesity

Reported success rates for treatment of childhood obesity are low. Successful management is greatly dependent on parents' attitude.

Parents must recognise the need for a child to become thinner, must be sufficiently motivated to make and sustain changes to the child's diet and if necessary that of the family, and be able to provide adequate emotional support for the child.

22.7.1   Management objectives

(1)   Prevent further weight gain until height has caught up in proportion to weight
(2)   Establish more appropriate eating habits
(3)   Increase physical activity

Treatment approaches must be age-dependent. In the family of a young child the focus should be on parental food purchasing and preparation as well as exercise activities.

Dietary modifications should take into account current diet, social circumstances and family income. Frequent reinforcement and *long-term* support are always necessary in order to maintain motivation.

22.7.2   Dietary modifications

Restrictive low-calorie diets are not suitable for young children because they may compromise dietary balance and ultimately growth adequacy. Parents should be advised against imposing such diets.

A suitable diet to slow weight gain in proportion to height is one which is low(er) in fat, low in sugar, contains plenty of fruit and vegetables and is adequate in respect of energy and other nutrients essential for growth.

What practical advice can I give?
Advice should be targeted at individual families but the following general suggestions may be helpful.

(1)   Reduce intake of foods high in sugar and/or fat. These snacks provide a lot of 'empty' calories. See alternative snack suggestions in Section 23.3.
(2)   Keep crisps, sweets and high sugar foods for special occasions only.
(3)   Cut down on sugar-containing drinks. These are high in calories and bad for teeth.
(4)   Give vegetables at each meal. Vary the choice and give them raw or cooked.

(5) Give semi-skimmed instead of whole milk. Give 280–560 ml ($\frac{1}{2}$–1 pint) per day to ensure a good calcium intake.
(6) Avoid frying foods; grill, bake or microwave instead.
(7) Give potatoes, rice, pasta or bread instead of chips at meal times.
(8) Give fruit each day – fresh, stewed or tinned in natural juice.
(9) Pay attention to portion sizes.

These guidelines can appear daunting. The most important points to get across are:

(1) Cut down on snacks and drinks between meals
(2) Serve more fruit and vegetables.
(3) Limit chips and fried foods

What about exercise?
This may include regular physical exercise such as swimming or walking to the shops, but any kind of active play such as nursery school

Table 22.1 Sample menu for 3–5 year old.

Breakfast	Lower sugar cereal, e.g. Weetabix, Shreddies, Rice Krispies with semi-skimmed milk and no sugar. Chopped fruit or raisins added to cereal if wished. One slice of bread or toast with small amount of spread. Milk or diluted fresh fruit juice.
Snack	Plain cracker or piece of fruit or raw vegetable sticks. Water or sugar-free squash.
Lunch	Roll, bread or toast with small amount of spread and filled, for instance, with tuna, meat, egg, baked beans. Vegetables – cooked or as a salad. Fruit or low fat yoghurt.
Snack	Fruit or handful of raisins, or one slice of bread or cracker. Water or sugar-free squash.
Evening meal	Meat, fish, egg or pulse dish. Vegetables or salad. Potato, rice or pasta. Fruit (tinned, cooked or fresh) or low fat yoghurt or fromage frais.
Bedtime	Milk drink (unsweetened).

games or 'helping' with housework will increase energy expenditure. Encouraging activity and exercise from an early age not only helps to build good habits but also provides an important means of socialising.

22.7.3   Psychological considerations

The psychological impact of limiting a child's food intake should not be underestimated. Too much emphasis on diet in front of an over-weight child can lead to a feeling of victimisation and resentment. It is very difficult to be denied favourite foods when others are seen to be allowed them. Changing the whole family's eating pattern is always preferable to individual restriction. Social eating situations, e.g. at nursery schools, with relatives or friends, need to be addressed without isolating the child. A child must not feel that he is being punished for being overweight, and encouragement and support is therefore crucial. Teasing (from adults or children) should not be tolerated.

Encourage parents to make things easier for the child. Advice might include the following:

At meal times

- Give the same meal as the rest of the family (see above)
- Give smaller portions
- Do not demand that food is finished, but do not give snacks in replacement
- Allow the child to become aware of being hungry. (This is often prevented by constant snacking)
- Serve favourite lower calorie foods, e.g. grilled fish fingers, baked beans

Shopping

- Walk to shops whenever possible
- Limit purchase of 'restricted' foods
- Encourage the child to 'help' with choosing items
- Avoid supermarket checkouts with sweet stands
- Do not give in to requests for sweets
- Avoid shopping when hungry

Socially

- Explain the need for restraint to grandparents, friends etc.; stress that the wellbeing of the child is at stake.

- Do not deny favourite foods entirely, but establish rules for when they are allowed
- Do not be over-concerned about special occasions, e.g. parties

Dietary changes are central to helping a child to lose weight, but these must be backed up by increased physical activity and broad social support. Changes need to be long-term.

Should an overweight child be referred to a dietitian?
All children with morbid obesity should be referred to a dietitian (see below). In cases of simple obesity, a child should be referred if:

- There is concern about the nutritional balance of the child's diet
- Simple weight maintenance advice has had little effect and parents are excessively anxious
- Weight is continuing to increase

Morbid obesity
Morbid obesity is rare in childhood and is most commonly associated with Prader-Willi Syndrome. This congenital disorder is associated with early feeding difficulties and then insatiable appetite from around 2–3 years.

All children with Prader-Willi Syndrome require specialist management and should be referred to a dietitian.

For further information contact the Prader-Willi Association, 2 Wheatsheaf Close, Harsell, Woking, Surrey, GU21 4BP.

22.8 Summary

Childhood obesity is common in Britain and reflects an energy intake in excess of requirements for growth. Weight in infancy is not related to adult obesity, but excessive weight gain in pre-school years may increase risk of adult obesity and is therefore to be avoided. Obesity is the result of interaction between genetic and environmental factors. Modification of eating habits is central to treatment and prevention of overweight in childhood and should start with a reduction of energy-rich snack foods. Low calorie diets are not suitable for young children since they may compromise nutrient needs for growth. Dietary modification should seek an increase in activity level, and strong family support is required for all overweight children.

23. Meals and Snacks

> 'There are many ways to get a good diet into young children. It just takes a bit of ingenuity, calmness and common sense.'
>
> Green, 1992

This chapter covers:

- The nutritional significance of breakfast, main meals and snacks
- Low-sugar snacks which can be given to young children
- Where to find information on menu-planning and simple meal suggestions

Providing a healthy family diet can be fraught with difficulty. The following are simple ideas for meals, snacks and drinks which are nutritionally appropriate for young children. Many are based on convenience foods. Recipe books giving more comprehensive suggestions are listed in the Resources Section. Meals are described in terms of food group choices. Reference to Chapter 12 and Appendix II is recommended.

23.1 Breakfast

A breakfast meal should include: the foods shown in Table 23.1.

Young children are not suited to long periods without food, and breakfast is an important energy-providing meal. Breakfast cereals make a significant contribution to iron intake and are to be encouraged. The provision of vitamin C rich fruit or diluted unsweetened fruit

Table 23.1 Foods that should be included in breakfast.

Food group	Food group symbol	Minimum servings
Bread, cereals and potatoes	B	1
Fruit and vegetables	F/V	1
Milk and dairy foods	M	1
Meat, fish and alternatives	M/A	Optional

juice will maximise iron absorption. Any variety of bread can be given
and bread alternatives such as muffin, roll, teacake, oatcake are also
suitable. Cooked foods (grilled bacon, baked beans etc.) are a useful
way of boosting the intake of faddy eaters who are unwilling to eat
breakfast.

Table 23.2 gives example breakfast menus for 4–5 year olds.

Table 23.2 Breakfast menu examples for age 4–5 years.

Food	Food Group Symbol
Weetabix with milk	B, M
White toast with spread	B
Diluted, unsweetened orange juice	F/V
Rice Krispies with milk	B, M
Toasted currant bread with spread	B
Satsuma	F/V
Grilled bacon	M/A
Wholemeal toast with spread	B
Pear slices	F/V
Milk to drink	M

23.1.1 Breakfast questions

Are high fibre cereals recommended?
No, not all varieties; bran and high fibre bran cereals are excessively
bulky, can cause diarrhoea and should not be given. Muesli is also
bulky and many varieties contain whole nuts which are not recommended for young children. Cereals such as Weetabix and Shredded
Wheat are perfectly acceptable.

What should be spread on bread?
A thin spreading of butter or margarine; additional options include
jam/reduced sugar jam, marmalade, honey, smooth peanut butter,
Marmite, cottage cheese, cheese spread, mashed banana. Low fat
spreads should not be used routinely.

Which fruits are high in vitamin C?
All citrus fruits and unsweetened citrus fruit juices, kiwi fruit and
melon are particularly high in vitamin C, but any kind of fruit,

including fruit tinned in unsweetened juice and dried fruit, is to be encouraged. Unsweetened fruit juice is acidic to dental enamel and, if given, should be diluted with at least equal parts water.

What about children who refuse to eat breakfast?
This is common. Suggest offering less traditional breakfast food as a substantial mid-morning snack such as:

- Milk, natural yoghurt and banana blended to a shake
- Fruit scone, margarine and a cup of milk
- Cheese triangle, plain crackers and diluted, unsweetened orange juice

23.2   Meals

A middle of the day and early evening meal should include:

Food group symbol	Minimum servings
B	1
F/V	1
M	1
M/A	1

The benefits of regular meals for pre-school children are described elsewhere (see Chapter 19). Meals do not have to be cooked meals, but choosing foods from each of the food groups encourages an adequate daily intake of all nutrients. Meal menus are listed here as cooked meals, convenience meals and sandwich meals. There is much overlap between these groups.

23.2.1   Cooked meals

Families' perceptions of a cooked meal differ greatly. High fat, high sugar meals are as unsuitable for pre-school children as they are for adults. Table 23.3 shows examples of suitable cooked meals.

23.2.2   Convenience food meals

Convenience foods have acquired a poor reputation, but foods which offer convenience do not have to be of low nutritional value. Eggs,

Table 23.3 Examples of suitable cooked meals.

Food	Food group symbol
Shepherds pie	M/A, B
Carrots	F/V
Stewed plums	F/V
Custard	M
Fish in cheese sauce	M/A, M
Boiled potato	B
Broccoli	F/V
Apple crumble	F/V
Chicken casserole	M/A
Rice	B
Sweetcorn	F/V
Banana custard	F/V, M

milk, tinned pulses, fruit are all 'convenience' foods. In general, less highly processed foods are the best choices. The convenience foods shown in Table 23.4 can be highly nutritious. Table 23.5 shows examples of convenience food menus. See Recommended Reading section for books with further suggestions.

Table 23.4 Examples of nutritious convenience foods.

Tinned	Fruit in natural juice, vegetables, pasta in sauce, soup, milk pudding, beans, fish
Dried	Instant potato, savoury rice with vegetables
Frozen	Vegetables, fish products, chicken nuggets, turkey/beef burgers, potato shapes, pizza
Chilled	Cooked meats, burgers, pizza bases, yoghurt, fromage frais

23.2.3 Sandwich meals

Sandwiches can fulfil all the nutritional criteria of a meal and are well-suited to children's needs. Cutting them into shapes increases their appeal and the number of possible sandwich combinations is limitless. For meal time sandwiches, one item should be selected from the examples listed in Table 23.6. Table 23.7 shows examples of menus for sandwich meals.

Table 23.5 Convenience food menus.

Food	Food group symbol
Fish fingers	M/A, B
Frozen peas	F/V
Alphabet potato letters	B
Fruit yoghurt	M
Baked beans	M/A
Toast with spread	B
Banana	F/V
Tinned pasta in sauce mixed with tinned vegetables and chopped ham	M/A
	F/V
Tinned peaches in unsweetened juice	F/V
Natural fromage frais	M

Can mayonnaise be used in sandwiches?

Yes, if it is bought mayonnaise. Home-made mayonnaise made from raw eggs should not be given to children under two years because of the potential risk of salmonella bacteria infection.

Is anything else unsafe?

Cheese made from unpasteurised milk should not be given to children under two years due to the risk of listeria infection. Tinned fish should always be checked for bones.

Table 23.6 Examples of meal time sandwiches.

Type of bread	Filling	Salad
Granary	Hard type cheese	Lettuce
Mighty White	Cheese slices/spread	Cucumber
White	Cottage Cheese	Grated carrot
Wholemeal	Smooth peanut butter	Tomato
Multigrain	Mashed baked beans	Raw courgette
Brown	Chickpea spread	Cress
Currant	Fish/meat paste	Raw mushroom
Pitta	Corned beef	Beansprouts
Roll	Cold meat	Raisins
Bap etc.	Mashed tinned fish	Banana etc.
	Chicken	
	Hard boiled egg	
	Vegetable pâté etc.	

Table 23.7 Examples of sandwich meal menus.

Food	Food group symbol
Egg and cress bap	M/A, B
Green salad	F/V
Fruit fromage frais	FN, M
Brown bread	B
Peanut butter, lettuce	M/A
Carrot sticks	F/V
Satsuma	F/V
White bread	B
Edam cheese	M
Tomato	F/V
Fruit yoghurt	M

23.3 Snacks

Snacks can make an important contribution to a child's daily nutrient intake, but should not decrease appetite for the next meal. Snacks should be low in NME sugars because frequent intake of NME sugars greatly increases risk of dental decay.

Snack suggestions

Best choices, low in NME sugars, are shown in Table 23.8. Other choices, containing more NME sugars and/or fat, are given in Table 23.9.

The following unsuitable snacks are high in NME sugars and of low nutritional value. If given, these foods should be offered immediately after meals:

- Chewy sweets
- Chocolate bars/sweets
- Chocolate and sweet biscuits
- Chewy muesli bars
- Sweet cakes and pastries

What about sugar-free sweets?

These are not recommended for everyday consumption. Sugar free sweets do not increase risk of tooth decay but do reinforce a preference for sweet foods. A high intake of sorbitol from such foods can cause diarrhoea.

Table 23.8 Snacks low in NME sugars.

Suggestion	Comments
Natural yoghurt Natural fromage frais }	Add chopped fruit, raisins, grated carrot, rolled oats
Raw vegetables Fresh fruit }	Give manageable portions
Bread, roll, toast	Any variety with spread or other if wished
Sandwiches	Any, see Section 23.2.3
Melba toast	Made by drying thinly cut bread in the oven
Bread sticks Oatcake Rice cake Krisp roll Plain cracker biscuits Crumpet Cheese scone }	With spread or other if wished
Cheese triangle/slice Plain popcorn	
Twiglets	High salt content

Table 23.9 Snacks containing more NME sugars.

Snack choice	Comments
Lower sugar cereal (optional: milk)	E.g. Shreddies, Rice Krispies
Plain/fruit scone Drop scone Currant bread Tea cake }	Most commercial varieties contain sugar
Plain sweet biscuits	
Cheesy biscuits Crisps Other savoury snacks }	Not for every day
Dried fruit	Sticky to teeth, therefore increased cariogenicity

23.4 Drinks

All drinks except water and milk can cause tooth decay and, if given, should be kept for meal times. Table 23.10 considers popular pre-school drinks.

Table 23.10 Suitability of popular drinks.

Drink	Comments
Water	Best choice.
Flavoured water	Some brands contain fructose which is cariogenic; check labels. Tap water can be flavoured by the addition of orange slices.
Bottled water	Acceptable after one year if parents concerned about water quality.
Carbonated mineral water	Not harmful to teeth, but filling for small stomachs.
Unsweetened fruit juice	Excellent source of vitamin C but acidic to dental enamel. Keep for meal times if possible. Dilute with a minimum of equal parts water.
Fruit juice concentrate	Available from health food shops, some supermarkets. Can be a cheaper way of buying fruit juice. *Must* be very well diluted, according to bottle instructions or more. Treat as fruit juice.
Ready to drink fruit drinks, e.g. Five-alive, Ribena	Contain sugar as well as fruit juice, therefore cariogenic. Give only at meal times, preferably diluted as above.
Reduced sugar fruit drinks, e.g. Ribena-light	May contain some sugar (sucrose) or sugar in another form; check labels. (The various forms of sugar are listed in Section 10.4.4.)
Diluting squash drinks	Contain high levels of sugar. Dilute very well. Give only at meal times.
Sugar-free squash drinks	Non-cariogenic. Sweetened with variety of artificial sweeteners. Can be used in moderation.
Carbonated drinks, e.g. Coca-Cola, Fanta, lemonade	Highly cariogenic due to sugar and acid content; **not advised.**
Diet drinks	Sugar-free, but acidic. If drunk frequently can damage tooth enamel (HEA, 1992); **not advised.**

Continued

Table 23.10 Continued.

Drink	Comments
Toddler fruit juice/ drinks	Some brands are vitamin fortified. May be less acidic than regular fruit juice but still potentially damaging to tooth enamel. Require dilution.
Milk	Good choice; plain milk is of low cariogenicity.
Flavoured milk drinks (including toddler milk drinks)	Often have a high sugar content except for Toddler brands which may also be vitamin fortified. May encourage a reluctant child to drink milk, but should only be given at meal times.
Yoghurt drinks	High sugar content (see above). Home-made versions preferable, i.e. yoghurt + milk + fruit.
Commercial milk shakes/powder	Very high sugar content. Keep for occasional meal times only. Very filling; may be consumed to the detriment of other food. Home-made versions preferable.
Herbal drinks	Check for added sugar.
Herbal teas	May be given over one year, e.g. mixed fruit, hibiscus varieties, cooled. Non-cariogenic. Do not give comfrey tea.
Soya milk, flavoured soya milk	Lower calcium content than cows' milk. Flavoured varieties generally contain sugar. Not recommended, unless chosen for dietary reasons. Young children drinking only soya milk may require calcium supplements.
Tea, coffee	Tannin in tea, and caffeine in tea and coffee, may inhibit iron absorption. Not recommended. If parents insist, ensure drink is weak, milky and without sugar.

Any discussion of pre-school drinks should include key points about good drinking habits:

- Give drinks from a cup or beaker
- Keep sweetened drinks for meal times
- Never give sweetened drinks before bed
- Remember that unsweetened fruit juice is acidic; give diluted with at least equal parts water
- Remember that drinks claiming 'no added sugar' often contain sugar in another form

See Chapter 10 for comprehensive dental health advice.

24. Additives

> 'Public concern about food additives is enhanced by a large amount of misinformation.'
>
> David, 1993

This chapter covers:

- Why additives are used in food
- The meaning of the term 'E number'
- Additives most commonly implicated in adverse reactions
- Reasons why diets high in additives are not recommended for children

The subject of additives continues to be a source of concern to many parents. The following is a brief account of common concerns. Further information about both Additives and Food Labelling is available from 'Food Sense' (see Resource List at the back of the book).

Why are additives used?
Additives are added to food for one of three purposes:

(1) To preserve food
(2) To modify consistency and texture.
(3) To enhance colour and/or flavour

The range of additives in existence, and the extent of their use, is a matter of some debate, but additives do allow access to a wider range of foods than would otherwise be possible.

Are additives safe?
There is no such thing as an absolute guarantee of safety. Even nutrients essential to life, e.g. zinc, copper, vitamin A, are toxic if consumed in huge quantities. When the safety of an additive is assessed, both the potential toxicity of the substance itself and the cumulative effect of long-term intake in an average diet are considered. An accepted daily intake (ADI) is then set, based on mg additive per kg

body weight. ADIs exist for most food additives in use, except flavourings, which are not subject to regulation at present. Whilst the ADI calculation is a guide to safe intake levels, toxicology is not an exact science and it is acknowledged that safety tests can produce conflicting results.

Also, little is known about the possible risks of interaction between different additives and it is very difficult to assess the possible long-term effect of a high additive intake (see Section 24.3.1).

24.1   The E number system

The E number system was devised as a means of labelling additives permitted for use in the European Union (EU) without reference to their full chemical name. Different sets of numbers have been allocated to different categories of additives. For example, colourings are numbered from E100 to E199. Any additive with an E number is approved for use in the EU. An additive number without an E prefix indicates that the additive is approved for use in the UK, but is not fully evaluated for use in the EU.

24.2   Additives and young children

Many additives are banned from use in baby foods because they are not needed or their possible effect on infants is unknown. Toddlers and pre-school children, however, may eat a wide range of additive-containing foods, e.g. soft drinks, crisps and confectionery, on a regular basis. Concern about additives and young children is commonly focused on the risk of additives provoking adverse reactions, but the lack of knowledge about high intakes at this age and the long-term toxicity, is possibly a greater cause for concern.

24.3   Adverse reactions to additives

It is now recognised that a small percentage of individuals do seem to be sensitive to specific additives, but a child is unlikely to be sensitive to additives alone.

The additives which are most commonly implicated in provoking adverse reactions are given in Table 24.1. Symptoms of intolerance include skin rashes (most common), respiratory problems, migraine, and, controversially, behavioural problems.

Table 24.1 Adverse reactions to additives.

Additive	E Number
Artificial colours (azo, coal tar, erythrosine dyes)	E102–E155
Natural colour: Annatto	E160b
Benzoate preservatives	E210–E219
Sulphur dioxide preservatives	E220–E224
Nitrite preservatives	E249–E252
Antioxidants BHA and BHT	E320–E321

From: Shaw & Lawson 1994. (Reproduced with permission.)

How common are adverse reactions?

The exact incidence of intolerance to additives is unknown but it is estimated to be very low, in the region of 0.01% to 0.23% of the population (Young *et al.*, 1987; MAFF, 1991). This figure is disputed by organisations such as the Hyperactive Children's Support Group, which believes the true incidence to be much higher.

24.3.1 Additives and hyperactivity

Behavioural problems or hyperactivity are commonly attributed to dietary additives. Hyperactivity is a term which is poorly defined and the term 'attention deficit disorder with hyperactivity' (ADDH) is preferable.

What causes ADDH?

It is generally believed that genetic, not environmental, factors are the cause of a tendency to ADDH. This tendency may then be exacerbated by environmental factors, e.g. disorganised lifestyle, poor parent-child interaction. Dr Ben Feingold first suggested a relationship between diet and behaviour in the 1970s (Feingold, 1975), but the association between diet and ADDH is highly controversial.

Studies since the 1970s have found evidence to suggest that there is a possible relationship between food and behaviour (Egger *et al.*, 1985; Kaplan *et al.*, 1989) but few hyperactive children have been found to respond to the elimination of food additives from their diet (David, 1987). Behavioural improvement resulting from additive free diets may be due in part to the more structured lifestyle associated with dietary restriction.

Although food additives may adversely affect hyperactive children, other foods can also do so. The most common foods producing adverse effects in susceptible children are those foods which generally cause food intolerance.

An elimination diet must always be prescribed and supervised by a paediatrician and a dietitian. Otherwise there is considerable risk of nutritional inadequacy.

What can I advise about additives and behaviour?
Parents should be made aware of the *very weak* association between additives and hyperactive behaviour. Strategies to organise a child's life are often a more appropriate means of tackling behavioural problems than dietary manipulation. Daily routines are to be encouraged.

If a lot of processed food is eaten, suggestion may be made to avoid those additives most commonly implicated in adverse reactions (see Table 24.1). Written information on additives is likely to be useful and can be obtained from a dietitian.

General diet-related advice is to:

- Cut down on processed foods, e.g. dessert mixes, flavoured crisps, chocolate and sweets, coloured squash drinks, packet sauce mixes, meat products
- Check labels for implicated additives wherever possible
- Look for foods with no added colouring

Avoidance of these food additives is unlikely to have nutritional implications, but parents must be cautioned against attempting any other form of dietary restriction without medical and dietetic advice (see above).

Is a diet high in additives harmful for children?
It can be if foods high in additives are eaten in place of more nutritious foods. Many high additive foods are low in vitamins and minerals.

On the present evidence, there is little reason to doubt that the majority of additives in current use are safe when consumed at normal dietary levels. A high intake of additives, unlike that of fat or sugar, has *not* been implicated as causative of chronic disease but given the lack of information relating to long-term additive intake, caution is prudent in respect of young children's diets. It is now not difficult for a young child to exceed the ADI for certain additives such as artificial sweeteners.

Artificial sweeteners are being used increasingly as a replacement for sugar in a wide range of foods and as a flavouring or flavour enhancer in others. Many foods containing artificial sweeteners are eaten regularly by young children. These include crisps and potato snacks, standard and diet type diluting drinks and fizzy drinks, sugar-free desserts and confectionery.

Example 1: Saccharine

ADI for saccharin	= 5 mg/kg
For a 3 year old child of 14 kg: ADI = 14 × 5	**= 70 mg**
3 glasses of standard orange drink	= 48 mg
1 can of diet fizzy drink	= 26 mg
1 portion of sugar-free dessert	= 15 mg
Total saccharine	**89 mg**

ADI is exceeded by 19 mg.

Example 2: Aspartame

ADI for Aspartame	= 40 mg/kg
For a 3 year old child of 14 kg: ADI = 14 × 40	= 420 mg
1 can of diet drink	= 198 mg
1 portion of sugar-free dessert	= 150 mg
1 portion of sugar-free baked beans	= 47 mg
1 sugar-free yoghurt	= 125 mg
Total Aspartame	520 mg

ADI is exceeded by 100 mg

What can I advise?
A moderate approach is recommended. There is no harm in young children eating some high additive foods as part of a mixed diet. Equally, there is no basis for being alarmist about sweeteners. Their use in some products, e.g. sugar-free squash, may benefit young children's teeth. Very high intakes of artificially sweetened foods are not recommended.

General advice
- Remember foods high in additives may be low in important nutrients, so restrict them.

- Avoid giving diet type carbonated drinks. These contain a lot of artificial sweeteners and their acid content is harmful to tooth enamel despite being sugar-free.
- Do not routinely use artificially sweetened products at meal times. Sugar in food given at meal times poses little risk to teeth.
- Remember artificially sweetened foods reinforce a preference for sweet foods. An oatcake is a better substitute for sugary confectionery than sugar-free sweets.

24.4 Summary

Additives are added to food to perform a specific, non-nutritive function. Additives are classified numerically according to their function and an E prefix indicates the substance is approved for use in the EU. Adverse reactions to additives are uncommon and rarely result in behaviour disturbance. The safety of additives in an average adult diet is not in doubt, but a high intake of artificially sweetened or other additive-rich foods is not recommended for children.

References and Further Reading for Section 3

Cole, T.J., Freeman, J. V. & Preece, M.A. (1995) Body mass index reference curves for the UK, 1990. *Arch. Dis. Child.*, 73, 25–9.

Cole-Hamilton, I. & Lang, T. (1986) Tightening Belts. *London Food Commission Report No. 13*, London.

David, T.J. (1987) Reactions to dietary tartrazine. *Arch. Dis. Child.*, 62, 119–22.

David, T.J. (1993) *Food and Food Additive Intolerance in Childhood*. Blackwell Science Ltd, Oxford.

DoH (1991) Department of Health Dietary Reference Values for Food, Energy and Nutrients for the United Kingdom. *Report on Health and Social Subjects No. 41*. HMSO, London.

DoH (1994) Department of Health Nutritional aspects of cardiovascular disease. *Report on Health and Social Subjects No. 46*. HMSO, London.

Egger, J., Carter, C.M., Graham, P.J., Gumley, D. & Soothill, J.F. (1985) Controlled trial of oligoantigenic treatment in hyperkinetic syndrome. *Lancet*, 1, 540–45.

Evans, D.J. & Dowell, J.B. (1991) The dental caries experience of 5 year old children in Great Britain. *Comm. Dental Health*, 8, 185–94.

Feingold, B.F. (1975) *Why Your Child is Hyperactive?* Random House, New York.

Finney, J. (1986) Preventing common feeding problems in infants and young children. *Pediatric Clinics of N. America*, 33, 4.

Fischer, R., Griffin, F., England, F. & Garn, F.M. (1961) Taste thresholds and food dislike. *Nature*, 191, 1328.

The Food Commission (1996) Cost of 100 kilocalories of various snack foods. Personal correspondence.

Francis, D. (1987) *Nutrition for Children*. Blackwell Science, Oxford.

Garrow, J.S. (1978) *Energy Balance and Obesity in Man*, 2nd edn. Elsevier, Amsterdam.

Green, C. (1992) *Toddler Training: a Parents Guide to the First Four Years*. Vermillion, London.

Gregory, J.R., Collins, D. L., Davies, P.S.W., Clark, P.C. & Hughes, J.M. (1995) *National diet and nutrition survey of children aged 1 and 4 years*. Office of Population, Census and Surveys. HMSO, London.

HEA (1992) *A Handbook of Dental Health for Health Visitors*. Health Education Authority, London.

Hollington, N. & Newby, C. (1995) Increasing cost of a healthy diet. *The Food Magazine*, 31, Oct./Dec.

Holt, R.D. (1990) Caries in the pre-school child. British Trends. *J.Dent.*, 18 269–99.

Holt, R.D., Joels, D., Bulman, J. & Maddick, I.H. (1988) A third study of caries in pre-school children in Camden. *Br. Dent. J.*, 165, 87–91.

James, J. (1992) Impact of low income on childhood diet. In *Nutrition, Social Status and Health*. Proceedings of a conference held in 1991 (ed. J.L. Butriss). National Dairy Council, London.

Kaplan, B.J., McNicol, J., Conte, R.A. & Moghadam, H.K. (1989) Dietary replacement in preschool-aged hyperactive boys. *Pediatrics*, 83, 7–17.

Lawrence B. (1991) *How to Feed your Family for £5 a Day*. Thorsons, London.

Lawson, M. (1994) Nutrition in Childhood. In *Nutrition, Social Status and Health*. Proceedings of two conferences. National Dairy Council, London.

MAFF (1991) Food allergy and other unpleasant reactions to food. *A Guide from the Food Safety Directorate*. HMSO, London.

Mooney, C. (1990) Cost and availability of healthy food choices in a London Health District. *J. Hum. Nutr. Dietet.* 3, 111–20.

NCH (1991) *Poverty and Nutrition Survey*. National Children's Home, London.

Nelson, M. & Peploe, K. (1990) Construction of a modest but adequate food budget for households with two adults and one child: a preliminary investigation. *J. Hum. Nutr. Dietet.*, 3, 121–40.

Payne, J.A. & Belton, N.R. (1992a) Nutrient intake and growth in pre-school children I. Comparison of energy intake and sources of energy with growth. *J. Hum. Nutr. Dietet.*, 5, 15–26.

Payne, J.A. & Belton, N.R. (1992b) Nutrient intake and growth in pre-school children II. Intake of minerals and vitamins. *J. Hum. Nutr. Dietet.*, 5, 27–32.

Poskitt, E. (1991) Early diet, later obesity? *Br. Nutr. Bull.*, 16, 38–44.

RCP (1983) Black, D. (Chairman): Obesity. *J. Royal Coll. Phys.*, 17, 5–65.

Rolland-Cachera, M.F., Deheeger, M., Bellisle, F., Sempe, M., Guilloud-Bataille, M. & Patois, E. (1984) Adiposity rebound in children: a simple indicator for predicting obesity. *Amer. J. Clin. Nutr.*, 39, 129–35.

Scottish Office (1993) *The Scottish Diet: report of a working party to the Chief Medical Officer for Scotland*. Scottish Home and Health Department, Edinburgh.

Serdula, M.K., Ivery, D., Coates, R.J., Freedman, D.S., Williamson, D.F. & Byers, T. (1993) Do obese children become obese adults? A review of the literature. *Prev.Med.* 22, 167–77.

Shaw, V. & Lawson, M. (eds.) (1994) *Clinical Paediatric Dietetics*. Blackwell Science Ltd, Oxford.

Skuse, D. (1993) Identification and management of problem eaters. *Arch. Dis. Child.*, 69, 604–608.

Sooman, A. & Taggart, J. (1992) *The West of Scotland Twenty-07 Study: Price and Availability of a Selection of 'Healthy' and 'Unhealthy' Food Items in Two Localities in Glasgow City.* Medical Research Council Medical Sociology Unit, Working Paper No. 33.

Taitz, L.S. (1991) *Textbook of Paediatric Nutrition*, 3rd edn. Churchill Livingstone, Edinburgh.

Thomas, B. (ed.) (1994) *Manual of Dietetic Practice*, 2nd ed. Blackwell Science Ltd, Oxford.

White, E.M., Wilson, A.C., Greene, S.A., McCowan, C., Thomas, G.E., Cairns, A.Y. & Ricketts I.W. (1995) Body Mass Index Centile Charts to assess fatness of British children. *Arch.Dis.Child.*, 72, 38–41.

Young, E., Patel, S., Stoneham, M., Rona R. & Wilkinson, J.D. (1987) The prevalence of reaction to food additives in a survey population. *J. Royal Coll. Phys.*, 21, 241–71.

Further reading

Davidson, S. *et al.* (1988) *Human Nutrition and Dietetics*, 8th edn. Churchill Livingstone, Edinburgh.

HEA (1989) *Diet, Nutrition and Healthy Eating in Low Income Groups.* Health Education Authority, London.

Krondl, M., Coleman, P., Wade, J. & Milner, J. (1983) A twin study examining the genetic influence on food selection. *Hum. Nutr. Appl. Nutr.*, 37A, 143–7

MAFF (1989) Household Food Consumption and Expenditure. *Annual Report of the National Food Survey Committee.* Ministry of Agriculture, Fisheries and Food.

NDC (1993) *Making Sense of Food Profile, No.3.* Children aged 4–6 years. National Dairy Council, London.

Appendices

Appendix I. The Cycle of Ill Health

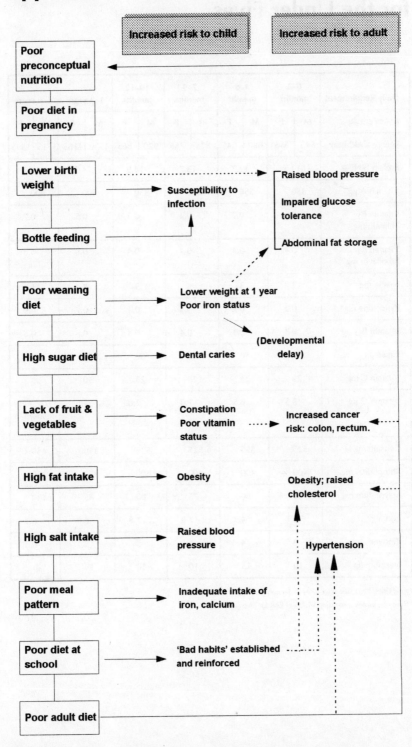

Appendix II. Dietary Reference Values for the Under Fives

Daily Requirement	0–3 months		4–6 months		7–9 months		10–12 months		1–3 years		4–6 years	
Male/Female	M	F	M	F	M	F	M	F	M	F	M	F
Energy (EAR) kcal	545	515	690	645	825	765	920	865	1230	1165	1715	1545
Protein (RNI) g	12.5		12.7		13.7		14.9		14.5		19.7	
Vitamin A µg	350		350		350		350		400		400	
Vitamin B$_1$ Thiamin mg	0.2		0.2		0.2		0.3		0.5		0.7	
Vitamin B$_2$ Riboflavin mg	0.4		0.4		0.4		0.4		0.6		0.8	
Niacin mg	3		3		4		5		8		11	
Pyridoxine mg*	0.2		0.2		0.3		0.4		0.7		0.9	
Vitamin B$_{12}$ µg	0.3		0.3		0.4		0.4		0.5		0.8	
Folate µg	50		50		50		50		70		100	
Vitamin C mg	25		25		25		25		30		30	
Vitamin D µg	8.5		8.5		7.0		7.0		7.0		0 if skin exposed to sun	
Calcium mg	525		525		525		525		350		450	
Phosphorus mg	400		400		400		400		270		350	
Magnesium mg	55		60		75		80		85		120	
Iron mg	1.7		4.3		7.8		7.8		6.9		6.1	
Zinc mg	4		4		5		5		5		6.5	
Selenium µg	10		13		10		10		15		20	

From: DoH, 1991 (see references to Section 3)

* Based on protein providing 14.7% of EAR for energy

Appendix III.   Welfare Food Scheme

The Welfare Food Scheme was introduced in 1940 to ensure that expectant mothers and young children were properly nourished. The scheme was retained after the war on the advice of the then standing committee on nutritional problems and it has continued to the present day with a number of modifications.

Expectant mothers and children under five years in families in receipt of Income Support receive the following, free of charge:

Welfare milk – 7 pints or 8 half litres of liquid milk per week. Infants under one year may receive instead 900 g per week of a range of specified brands of infant formula. Breastfeeding mothers may elect to take their baby's entitlement of infant formula in the form of liquid milk to drink themselves.

Vitamin supplements – Expectant mothers receive two bottles of vitamin drops or 90 tablets every 13 weeks for the duration of pregnancy. Breasfeeding mothers receive five bottles of drops or 225 tablets in total. Children under five receive two bottles of drops every 13 weeks. Both drops and tablets contain vitamins A, C and D (Table A1).

Table A1   Vitamin content of vitamin drops.

Department of Health vitamin drops (5 drops) contain:
• Vitamin A (retinol equivalents) 200 µg • Vitamin C 20 mg • Vitamin D$_3$ 7 µg

From: *Weaning and The Weaning Diet* (DoH, 1994 – see references to Section 2).

Parents of children aged under one year in families in receipt of Family Credit are entitled to purchase 900 g of infant formula per week from clinics at a reduced price.

Children aged under five years in the care of registered childminders and certain day care providers may receive one third of a pint of liquid milk (or for children aged under one year, infant formula made up to one third of a pint) for each day spent in day care.

Handicapped children aged over five years but under the age of 16 years who are not able to attend an educational establishment by reason of their disability, are entitled to 7 pints or 8 half litres of liquid milk free per week and to free vitamin supplements.

Liquid milk means whole or semi-skimmed liquid cow milk. Liquid milk is available under the Welfare Food Scheme from a wide range of shops and milk roundsmen.

Resources

Recommended Reading

Specific Reports

Early diet

Barker, D.J.P., Winter, P.D., Osmond, C., Margetts, B. & Simmonds, S.J. (1989) Weight in infancy and death from ischaemic heart disease. *Lancet*, **ii**, 577–80.

Bartley, M., Power, C., Blane, D., Davey Smith, G. & Shipley, M. (1994) Birthweight and later socio-economic disadvantage: evidence from the 1958 British Cohort Study. *B.M.J.*, 309, 1475–9.

Lucas, A. (1994) Role of nutritional programming in determining adult morbidity. *Arch.Dis.Child.*, 71, 288–90.

Lucas, A., Bishop, N.J., King, F.J. & Cole, T.J. (1992) Randomised trial of nutrition for preterm infants after discharge. *Arch.Dis.Child.*, 67, 324–7.

Nutrient intakes

Mills, A. (1993) Dietary survey of infants aged 6 to 12 months. *Nutrition and Food Science*, 3, 9–13.

Payne, J.A. & Belton, N.R. (1992) Nutrient intake and growth in pre-school children. I. Comparison of energy intake and sources of energy with growth. *J. Hum.Nutr.Dietet*, 5, 287–98.

Payne, J.A. & Belton, N.R. (1992) Nutrient intake and growth in pre-school children. II. Intake of vitamins and minerals. *J.Hum.Nutr.Dietet.*, 5, 27–32.

Scower, P. (1993) Infant feeding in the UK: birth to nine months. How British babies are fed. *Professional Care of the Mother and Child*, 3(9) 256–7.

Growth

Hindmarsh, P.C. & Brook, C.G.D. (1994) Measuring the growth of children in general practice. *Maternal and Child Health*, June.

Marcovitch, H. (1994) Failure to thrive. *B.M.J.*, 308, 35–38.

Knowledge

Hyde, L. (1994) Knowledge of basic infant nutrition amongst community health professionals. *Maternal and Child Health*, Jan., 27–32.

Ko, M.L.B., Ramsell, N. & Wilson, J.A. (1992) What do parents know about vitamins? *Arch.Dis.Child.*, 67, 1080–81.

Iron deficiency

Duggan, M. (1993) Cause and cure of iron deficiency in toddlers. *Health Visitor*, **66**(7) 250–52.

Grindulis, H., Scott, P.H., Belton, N.R. & Wharton, B.A. (1986) Combined deficiency of iron and vitamin D in Asian toddlers. *Arch.Dis.Child.*, **61**, 843–8.

Harbottle L. & Duggan, M.B. (1992) Comparative study of the dietary characteristics of Asian toddlers with iron deficiency in Sheffield. *J. Hum. Nutr. Dietet.*, **5**, 351–61.

Idjradinata, P., Watkins, W.E. & Pollitt, E. (1994) Adverse effect of iron supplementation on weight gain in iron replete young children. *Lancet*, **343**, 1252–4.

Mills, A.F. (1990) Surveillance for anaemia: risk factors in patterns of milk intake. *Arch.Dis.Child.*, **65**, 428–31.

Oski, F.A. (1993) Iron deficiency in infancy and childhood. *New Eng.J.Med.*, 15 July, 190–93.

Palmer, G. (1993) Weaning any old iron. *Health Visitor*, **66** (7) 248–9.

Asian

Gatrad, A.R., Birch, N. & Hughes, M. (1994) Pre-school weights and heights of Europeans and five subgroups of Asians in Britain. *Arch.Dis.Child.*, 207–10.

Jones, V.M. (1987) Current weaning practices within the Bangladeshi community in the London Borough of Tower Hamlets. *Hum.Nutr.Appl.Nutr.*, **41A**, 349–352.

Warrington, S. & Storey, D.M. (1988) Comparative studies on Asian and Caucasian children. 2: Nutrition feeding practices and health. *Eur. J.Clin.Nutr.*, **42**, 69–80.

Low income

Mooney, C. (1990) Cost and availability of healthy food choices in a London Health District. *J.Hum.Nutr.Dietet.*, **3**, 111–120.

Dental Health

Bentley, E. (1994) Views about preventive dental care for infants. *Health Visitor*, **67** (3) 88–9.

Dugal, M.S. & Curzon, M.E.J. (1989) An evaluation of the cariogenic potential of baby and infant food and drinks. *British Dental Journal*, 6 May 327–30.

Evans, D.J. & Dowell, J.B. (1991) The dental caries experience of five year old children in Great Britain. *Comm.Dental Health*, **8**, 185–94.

Lobstein, T. (1995) Baby drinks hazards. *Living Earth and the Food Magazine*, April/June.

Food allergy/intolerance

David, T.J. (1989) Dietary treatment of atopic eczema. *Arch.Dis.Child.*, **64**, 506–509.

Devlin, J., Stanton, R.H. & David T.J. (1989) Calcium intake and cows milk free diets. *Arch.Dis.Child.*, **64**, 1183–4.

General publications

Books

Barker, D.J.P (ed). (1992) *Fetal and Infant Origins of Adult Disease*. BMJ Books, London.

Barker, D.J.P. (1994) *Mothers, Babies and Diseases in Later Life*. BMJ Books, London.

Clayden, G. & Agnarsson, U. (1991) *Constipation in Childhood*. Oxford University Press, Oxford.

Hill, S.E. (1990) *More than Rice and Peas: Guidelines to Improve Food Provision for Black and Ethnic Minorities in London*. The London Food Commission, London.

Hull, S. (1992) *Safe Cooking for a Healthy Baby*. Penguin, London.

Lobstein, T. (1988) *Children's Food*. Unwin/The London Food Commission, London.

Palmer, G. (1988) *The Politics of Breast-feeding*. Pandora Press, London.

Royal College of Midwives. (1991) *Successful Breast-feeding* 2nd edn., Churchill Livingstone, Edinburgh.

Rugg-Gunn, A.J. (1993) *Nutrition and Dental Health*. Oxford University Press, Oxford.

Sahota, P. (1991) *Feeding Baby: Inner City Practice*. Horton Publishing, Bradford.

Salmon, J. (1991) *Dietary Reference Values: A Guide*. Department of Health, London.

Taitz, L.S. & Wardley, B.L. (1990) *Handbook of Child Nutrition*. Oxford Medical Publications, Oxford.

Whiting, M. & Lobstein, T. (1992) *The Nursery Food Book*. Hodder and Stoughton/The London Food Commission, London.

Reports

DoH (1991) Dietary Reference Values for Food Energy and Nutrients for the United Kingdom. *Report on Health and Social Subjects No. 41.* HMSO, London.

DoH (1994) Nutritional Aspects of Cardiovascular Disease. *Report on Health and Social Subjects No. 46.* HMSO, London.

DoH (1994) Weaning and the Weaning Diet. HMSO, London. *Report on Health and Social Subjects No. 45.* HMSO, London.

DHSS (1988) Present Day Practice in Infant Feeding. Third Report. *Report on Health and Social Subjects No. 32.* HMSO, London.

Gregory, J.R., Collins, D.L., Davies, P.S.W., Clark, P.C. & Hughes, J.M. (1995) *National Diet and Nutrition Survey of Children aged 1 to 4 years.* HMSO, London.

Mills, A. & Tyler, H. (1992) *Food and Nutrient Intakes of British Infants aged 6–12 months.* HMSO, London.

National Breastfeeding Working Group/Department of Health (1995) *Breastfeeding: Good Practice Guidance to the NHS.* DoH, London.

National Children's Home (1994) *Poverty and Nutrition Survey.* NCH, London.

White, A. *et al.* (1992) *Infant Feeding 1990.* HMSO, London.

Briefing Papers

Buttriss J. (ed) (1991) Nutrition, Social Status and Health. *Proceedings of the National Dairy Conference.* NDC, London.

Buttriss, J. & Hyman, K. (eds) (1991) Mother and Child. *Proceedings of the National Dairy Council Conference.* NDC, London.

HEA (1991) *Nutrition in Ethnic Minority Groups.* Health Education Authority, London.

HEA (1992) *A Handbook of Dental Health for Health Visitors.* Health Education Authority, London.

HEA (1996) *The Scientific Basis of Dental Health Education.* Health Education Authority, London.

Health Education Board for Scotland (HEBS) (1993) *The Food Hygiene Handbook for Scotland,* 7th edn. Highfield Publications, Doncaster.

National Dairy Council (1989) *Factfile 2: Nutrition and Children aged One to Five.* NDC, London.

National Dairy Council (1990) *Factfile 6: Nutrition and Vegetarianism.* NDC, London.

National Dairy Council (1994) *Factfile 11: Maternal and Fetal Nutrition.* NDC, London.

National Dairy Council, (1994) *Topical Update 3: Weaning and the Weaning Diet.* NDC, London.

Magazines/Journals

Archives of Diseases in Childhood
BBC Good Food Magazine
British Medical Journal
Health Visitor
Journal of Human Nutrition and Dietetics
The Lancet
Living Earth and the Food Magazine
NDC Quarterly Review
Nursing Times
Nutrition and Food Science
Which? Way to Health

Resource List: Organisations

W = written information: leaflets, reports, guidelines, briefing papers, updates etc.
A = advice: department within the organisation provides information.
PRO = professional resource: no access for the lay public.

Association of Breastfeeding Mothers *(W,A)*
PO Box 441
St Albans
Herts AL4 0AF
Tel: 0181 778 4769

British Dental Association *(W, A, PRO)*
64 Wimpole Street
London W1M 8AL
Tel: 0171 935 0875

British Dental Health Foundation *(W, A, PRO)*
Eastlands Court
St. Peters Road
Rugby CV21 3QP
Tel: 01788 546365

British Dietetic Association *(W, A, PRO)*
7th Floor, Elizabeth House
22 Suffolk Street, Queensway
Birmingham B1 1LS
Tel: 0121 643 5483

British Nutrition Foundation *(W, PRO)*
Holborn House
52–54 High Holborn
London WC1V 6RQ
Tel: 0171 404 6504

Castlemead Publications *(W, PRO)*
12 Little Mundells
Welwyn Garden City
Herts AL7 1EW
Tel: 01707 320 220

Child Growth Foundation *(W, PRO)*
2 Mayfield Avenue
Chiswick
London W4 1PW
Tel: 0181 995 0257

Community Practitioners Health Visitors Association *(W, A, PRO)*
50 Southward Street
London SE1 1UN
Tel: 0171 717 4000

English National Board for Nursing, Midwifery and Health Visiting *(W, PRO)*
Resource Section
Victory House
170 Tottenham Court Road
London W1P 0HA
Tel: 0171 388 3131

The Food Safety Advisory Centre *(W, A)*
Foodline
72 Rochester Row
London SW1P 1JU
Tel: 0800 282 407

Food Sense
(MAFF Food Safety Publications)
(W)
London SE99 7TP
Tel: 01645 556 000

HEA Resources *(W, PRO)*
HEA Customer Services
Marston Book Services
PO Box 269
Abingdon
Oxon OX14 4YN
Tel: 01235 465 565

Health Education Authority *(A, PRO)*
Hamilton House
Mabledon Place
London WC1H 9TX
Tel: 0171 383 3833
Information line: 0171 413 1995

Health Education Board for Scotland *(W, PRO)*
Woodburn House
Canaan Lane
Edinburgh
EH10 4SG
Tel: 0131 536 5500

Midwives Information & Resources Services (MIDIRS) *(W, PRO)*
9 Elmdale Road
Clifton
Bristol BS8 1SL
Tel: 0117 925 1791

National Childbirth Trust *(W, A)*
Alexandra House
Oldham Terrace
London W3 6NH
Tel: 0181 992 8637

National Dairy Council *(W, PRO)*
5–7 John Princes Street
London W1M 0AP
Tel: 0171 499 7822

The National Eczema Society *(W, A)*
163 Eversholt Street
London NW1 1BU
Tel: 0171 388 4097

The National Food Alliance *(W)*
5–11 Worship Street
London EC2A 2BH
Tel: 0171 628 2442

Royal College of Midwives *(W, A, PRO)*
15 Mansfield Street
London W1M OBE
Tel: 0171 872 5100

Twins & Multiple Births Association (TAMBA) *(W, A)*
PO Box 30
Little Sutton
South Wirral
L66 1PH
Tel: 0151 348 0020

UNICEF/Baby Friendly Initiative *(W, PRO)*
55 Lincolns Inn Fields
London WC2A 3NB
Tel: 0171 405 5592

The Vegetarian Society *(W, A)*
Parkdale, Dunham Road
Altrincham
Cheshire WA14 4QG
Tel: 0161 928 0793

Information Recommended for Patients

Leaflets

Association of Breastfeeding Mothers (Sample of publications available)
Have I Got Enough Milk?

British Dental Health Foundation
Dental Care for Mother and Baby
Preventive Care and Oral Hygiene

British Dietetic Association
Food for the Growing Years (1–5 year olds)

Food Safety Advisory Centre
The Good Food Safety Guide
Safe Food

Food Sense
Food Safety
About Food Additives
Food Allergy
Understanding Food Labels

Health Education Authority (Sample of publications available)
Breastfeeding: Your Questions Answered
Birth to Five Book
From Milk to Mixed Feeding

National Childbirth Trust (Sample of publications available)
Breastfeeding: Avoiding Some of the Problems
Breadfeeding: Returning to Work

National Dairy Council
A Guide for You and Your Baby
The Step by Step Guide to Weaning
Your Child and Milk
Healthy Eating Guide for the One to Fives

National Farmers' Union (NFU, 164 Shaftesbury Avenue, London
WC2H 8HL. Tel: 0171 331 7200)
Your Baby's First Vegetables

The Vegetarian Society
First Foods

Books

Consumers' Association (1988) *Understanding Food Additives*. Consumers'
  Association and Hodder and Stoughton, London.
Food Safety Advisory Centre (1993) *Food Safety: Questions and Answers*
  FSAC, London.
Green, C. (1993) *Toddler Training*. Vermilion, London.
Green, C. (1995) *Understanding Attention Deficit Disorder – a Parents' Guide
  to ADD in Children*. Vermilion, London.
Green, C. (1996) *Babies*. Simon and Schuster Ltd, London.
HEA (1991) *Birth to Five*. Health Education Authority, London.
Jackson, P. (1995) *Vegetarian baby and child*. Headline Book Publishing,
  London.
Karmel, K. (1995) *Annabel Karmel's Baby and Toddler Cookbook*. Ebury
  Press, London.
Kitzinger, S. (1989) *Breastfeeding your baby*. Dorling Kindersley, London.
Lawrence, B. (1991) *How to Feed your Family for £5.00 a Day*. Thorsons,
  London.
Morse, E. (1988) *My Child Won't Eat*. Penguin, London.
Renfrew, M. *et al.* (1990) *Breastfeeding*. Celestial Arts, California. Available
  through MIDIRS Book Service, Bristol.
Smale, M. (1992) *The NCT Book of Breastfeeding*. Vermilion, London.
Welford, H. (1994) *Feeding your Child from Birth to Three*. HEA, London.
Whiting, M. & Lobstein, T. (1995) *Teach yourself Healthy Eating for babies
  and children*. Hodder and Stoughton, London.

Index

additives, 219–24
Afro-Caribbean diets, 171–2
allergy, *see* food intolerance and allergy
aluminium, soya formula, 76
antimicrobial factors, 7
appetite, 150
artificial sweeteners, 54, 222–4
Asian diets, 168–71
attention deficit disorder, 221–2

bottle feeding, 20–26
  Asian practice, 170
  casein dominant milk, 21, 22–4
  changing milks, 23–4, 29
  colic, 29
  constipation, 27–8
  cow's milk, 69–73
  ewe's milk, 59, 74–5
  feed preparation, 24–5
  follow-on milk, 73–4, 77
  goat milk formula, 74
  goat's milk, 59, 74
  infant milk composition, 5–6, 21–3, 30, 40
  infant milk marketing, 25–6
  low birth weight infants, 39, 40
  microwave ovens, 25
  nutrient enriched milks, 40
  refusal to stop, 155–6
  soya formula, 23, 75–6, 85–6
  soya 'milk', 76
  supplementing breast milk, 17–18
  trends, 20–21
  vegan infants, 59

vitamin supplements, 30, 31
weaning diet, 77
whey dominant milk, 21, 22, 23–4
bowel problems, 27–8, 157–60
breakfast, pre-school, 210–12
breastfeeding, 3–19
  additional fluids, 16
  advantages, 8, 18
  Afro-Caribbean practice, 171
  antimicrobial factors, 7
  Asian practice, 170
  carbohydrates, 5
  colic, 29
  colostrum, 3
  composition of milk, 3–4
  constipation, 27
  contraindications, 18
  establishment, 15–16
  failure to thrive, 16–17
  fat content, 4–5
  fatty acids, 5–6
  food intolerance, 14, 29, 82
  growth factors, 7
  intervention strategies, 19
  length of, 10
  low birth weight infants, 39–40
  maintenance, 15–16
  maternal diet, 10–14, 29, 82, 84–5, 233
  milk production, 6, 8
  minerals, 5
  non-food substances, 14
  posseting, 29
  promotion, 18–19
  protein concentration, 4

reasons for stopping, 9–10
refusal to stop, 155–6
supplementary feeds, 17–18
trends, 8–9
vitamins, 5, 12–13, 14, 30, 31
weaning diet, 77

calcium
Chinese diets, 172
dietary reference values, 232
lactating mothers, 12
pre-school children, 181
toddlers, 122, 130–31, 166–7
vegetarian diet, 166–7
Vietnamese diets, 172
Campylobacter, 106
carbohydrate, breast milk, 5
casein dominant milk, 21, 22–4
chewing, refusal, 155
Chinese diets, 172
coeliac disease, 50–51
colic, 29–30
colostrum, 3
constipation, 27–28, 158–60
convenience foods, 212–13
cooked meals, 212–13
cow's milk, 69–73
gastrointestinal blood loss, 70
infant milks from, 21–2
intolerance, 14, 70, 83–7
iron, 64, 70
lactating mothers, 14, 29
protein intolerance, 84, 87
recommended use, 71–2, 77
reduced fat, 72–3
renal solute load, 69–70
vitamin D, 70
weaning diet, 77

dental health, 88–98
Asian diet, 171

dental visits, 97
dietary sugars, 90–5
eating patterns, 184–5
fluoride, 95–6
low income diets, 193–4
plaque, 90
prevalence of caries, 88–9
primary dentition, 98
process of caries, 89
saliva, 89–90
soya formula, 75–6
sugar intake frequency, 90
sugar labelling, 95
teething, 98
toddler diet, and, 139–40
tooth brushing, 96–7
diarrhoea, toddlers, 157–8
dietary adequacy, 59–60, 125–35
Dietary Reference Values, 121–3,
232
dietary variety, 54–5, 56, 77, 198
diet history, toddlers, 127–9
drinks
additives, 223, 224
during weaning, 57
low income diets, 193
pre-school children, 217–18
sugar in, 92–4
see also fluid intake
drugs, lactating mothers, 14

eating habits, pre-school, 181–6
eating skills, toddlers, 143–5
elimination diets, infants, 81
energy intake
average requirements, 120,
121–2
dietary reference values, 232
food refusal, 150
lactating mothers, 11–12
low birth weight infants, 40, 42

pre-school children, 180
vegetarian toddlers, 163
vegetarian weaning, 58
E numbers, 220
Escherichia coli, 107
ethnic minority diets, 163,
168–73
evening meals, 212–16
ewe's milk, 59, 74–5
exclusion diets, 13–14, 29

faddiness, 196–201
failure to thrive, 16–17, 35–7
fat nutrition
breast milk, 4–6
cow's milk, 72–3
infant milks, 21
toddler diet, 137, 138
weaning foods, 55, 56
feeding problems
ending breast/bottle feeding,
155–6
faddiness, 196–201
food refusal, 77, 131, 149–54
refusing to chew, 155
vomiting on demand, 154–5
fibre, toddler diet, 123, 137–9
fluid intake
breastfed babies, 16
during weaning, 57
lactating mothers, 12
see also drinks
fluoride, dental health, 95–6
follow-on milk, 73–4, 77
food intolerance and allergy,
78–87
breastfeeding, 14, 29, 82
coeliac disease, 50–51
colic, 29
cow's milk, 14, 70, 83–7
definitions, 78

diagnosis, 81
environmental factors, 83
ewe's milk, 75
foods causing, 79
goat's milk, 74
maternal diet, 14, 82, 84–5
prevalence, 79–80
reactions to food, 79
risk factors, 81–3
symptoms, 80
weaning, 51, 82–3
food poisoning, *see* food safety
food refusal, 149–54
causes, 149–51
faddiness, 196–201
management, 151–4, 198–9
meat, 199–200
milk in pre-school diet, 201
milk in toddler diet, 131
milk in weaning diet, 77
vegetables, 200
see also meal times
food safety, 99–108
bottle feeding, 24, 25
causes of poisoning, 99–100
common micro-organisms,
105–107
cooking, 102, 103
frozen foods, 102, 103, 104
heating foods, 102
high risk foods, 104–105
kitchen hygiene, 101
mealtime hygiene, 101
microwave ovens, 25, 103,
104
reducing poisoning risk, 100–
103, 105, 106, 107
refrigeration, 101–102,
103–104
reheating food, 103
storage, 101–102, 103–104

gastro-oesophageal reflux, 28–9
gluten, weaning foods, 50–51
goat's milk, 59, 74
growth, 32–7
   Asian infants, 170
   assessment in toddlers, 127
   centile charts, 33–4, 41
   failure to thrive, 16–17, 35–7
   head circumference, 33, 35
   importance in infancy, 32
   linear, 34–5
   low birth weight infants, 41
   monitoring, 32–3
   velocity, 35
   weight measurement, 32–3, 34

head circumference, 33, 35
healthy eating
   ill health cycle, 231
   obesity, 204
   pre-school diet, 179–86
   toddlers, 136–42
   see also low income diets
height measurement, 32–3, 34–5,
   41
hydrolysed protein formula, 85
hygiene, *see* food safety
hyperactivity, 221–2

ill health cycle, 231
income, *see* low income diets
infant milks
   casein dominant, 21, 22–4
   changing, 23–4, 29
   composition, 5–6, 21–3, 30, 40
   follow-on milk, 73–4, 77
   goat milk formula, 74
   hydrolysed protein formula, 85
   low birth weight, 39, 40
   marketing, 25–6
   nutrient enriched, 40

   soya formula, 23, 75–6, 85–6
   vitamin supplements, 30, 31
   weaning diet, 77
   whey dominant, 21, 22, 23–4
infants
   bottle feeding, 20–26
   breastfeeding, 3–19
   colic, 29–30
   constipation, 27–8
   cow's milk, 69–73
   dental health, 88–98
   ethnic feeding practices,
     170–73
   ewe's milk, 59, 74–5
   follow-on milk, 73–4, 77
   food intolerance/allergy,
     78–87
   food safety, 99–108
   goat's milk, 59, 74
   growth, 32–7
   iron nutrition, 61–8
   low birth weight, 38–43
   obesity, 203
   posseting, 28–9
   soya formula, 23, 75–6, 85–6
   soya 'milk', 59, 76
   vitamin supplements, 30–31
   weaning, 44–60, 77
iron, 61–8, 123, 131–5
   absorption, 63–4
   Afro-Caribbean diet, 172
   Asian diet, 170
   assessment, 133–5
   breast milk, 4
   cow's milk, 64, 70
   deficiency prevalence, 61–2
   deficiency screening, 67–8
   follow-on milk, 73
   haem iron, 63
   lactating mothers, 13
   low birth weight, 41

low income diets, 190–92
non-haem iron, 63–4
pre-school children, 181,
    190–92
reasons for deficiency, 62, 132
requirements, 62, 232
supplements, 67
vegetarian, 58, 65, 67, 167
weaning foods, 55–6, 58, 61,
    64–6, 67

Jewish diets, 173

lactose, 4, 5, 91–2
    intolerance, 83–4, 87, 172–3
length measurement, 32–3, 34–5,
    41
Listeria, 105–106
low birth weight infants, 38–43
low income diets, 187–95
    characteristics, 187–8
    constraints, 188–90
    fruit intake, 192, 193
    iron intake, 190–92
    sugar intake, 193–4
    vegetable intake, 192
    Welfare Food Scheme, 233–4

maternal diet, 10–14, 29, 31, 82,
    84–5, 233
meals
    managing obesity, 207, 208
    pre-school, 182–3, 210–15
meal times, toddlers, 143–8
microwave ovens, 25, 103, 104
mid-day meals, 212–16
minerals
    breast milk, 4, 5
    dietary reference values, 232
    infant milks, 21
    lactating mothers, 13

low birth weight infants, 41
soya formula, 76
supplements, 31
toddlers, 123, 167
vegetarian diet, 167
weaning foods, 55–6, 58
see also iron

obesity, 202–209

phosphorus, 4, 232
phytoestrogens, soya formula,
    76
playing with food, 148
posseting, 28–9
poverty, *see* low income diets
Prader–Willi syndrome, 209
pre-school children
    additives, 219–24
    dietary reference values, 232
    drinks, 217–18
    faddiness, 196–201
    healthy eating, 179–86, 232
    low income diets, 187–95
    meals, 182–3, 210–15
    obesity, 202–209
    snacks, 183–4, 193, 194,
        215–16
presenting food, 145–6, 150,
    198
pre-term infants, 38–43
protein
    cow's milk, 69–70, 84, 87
    dietary reference values, 232
    in breast milk, 4
    infant milks, 21, 22
    lactating mothers, 12
    pre-school children, 180
    toddlers, 122, 165–6
    vegetarian diets, 58, 165–6
    weaning foods, 55, 58

protein hydrolysate, 85

refusing food, *see* food refusal
rickets, 170–71, 172
rotavirus infection, 107
Salmonella, 105
salt
   toddler diet, 140–42
   weaning foods, 49, 54, 56
sandwich meals, 213–15
semi-skimmed milk, 72–3
skimmed milk, 72–3
snacks, 183–4, 193, 194, 215–16,
   223–4
sodium, 4, 22
   see also salt
soya infant formula, 23, 75–6,
   85–6
soya 'milk', 59, 76
Staphylococcus, 106–107
sugar
   dental health, 89–95, 184–5
   labelling, 95
   low income diets, 193–4
   pre-school diet, 183, 184, 185,
      193–4, 215–16
   toddler diet, 139–40, 141
   weaning foods, 49–50, 54, 55,
      56

teeth, *see* dental health
toddlers
   constipation, 158–60
   diarrhoea, 157–8
   dietary adequacy, 125–35
   ethnic groups, 163, 168–73
   feeding problems, 149–56
   future health, 136–42
   meal times, 143–8
   nutritional needs, 119–24, 232
   obesity, 203

vegetarianism, 163–8
vitamin supplements, 160–62

vegan diets, 58–9, 164–8
vegetarianism, 57–9, 65, 67,
   163–8
Vietnamese diets, 172–3
vitamins
   Asian diet, 170–71
   breast milk, 4, 5, 13, 14, 31
   cow's milk, 70
   dietary reference values, 232
   ewe's milk, 75
   goat's milk, 74, 75
   infant milks, 21, 30, 31
   lactating mothers, 12–13, 14,
     31
   low birth weight infants, 41
   overdosing, 161–2
   pre-school children, 181
   supplements, 30–31, 41, 58,
     160–62, 233–4
   toddlers, 123, 160–62, 167,
     170–71
   vegetarian diet, 167
   Vietnamese diet, 173
   weaning foods, 55, 58–9
   Welfare Food Scheme, 233–4
vomiting on demand, 154–5

weaning, 44–60
   Afro-Caribbean practice, 171,
     172
   age of, 45–7
   Asian practice, 170
   at 4–6 months, 48–53
   at 6–9 months, 53–6
   at 9–12 months, 56–7
   constipation, 28
   convenience foods, 56–7
   dental health, 94–5

drinks during, 57
family foods, 56–7
food consistency, 48–9, 53–4,
    56
food flavour, 50
food intolerance, 51, 82–3,
    86–7
food quantity, 48, 53
food variety, 54–5, 56, 77
gluten, 50–51
home-made foods, 51–3, 56
iron nutrition, 55–6, 58, 61,
    64–6, 67
low birth weight infants, 41–3
manufactured foods, 51–3, 56
milk free, 86–7

nutritional adequacy, 59–60
purées, 48–9
reasons for, 44–5
refusal, 155–6
role of milk in, 77
salt, 49, 54, 56
sugar, 49–50, 54, 55, 56
vegetarian, 57–9, 65, 67
weight loss, maternal, 12
weight measurement, 32–3, 34
weight problem, obesity,
    202–209
welfare Food Scheme, 233–4
wellbeing assessment, 127
whey dominant milk, 21, 22,
    23–4